THE WASTI

A Critique of Infant & Child Nutrition

POLICY, PRACTICE & POLITICS

Stewart Forsyth

Published by Swan & Horn 2023
KDP paperback ISBN 9798852401526
Also available on Kindle.

Disclaimer: The information in this critique is based on the Author's knowledge and experience and reflects on the role of the key parties involved in infant and child nutrition, with the objective of being fair and reasonable, and the opinions expressed herein are those of the Author. The Author is not liable for any risks or issues associated with using or acting upon the information contained in this book, and it should not be misconstrued as advice for pregnant women, or infants and young children. Despite the concerted effort of the Author, there are no representations or warranties, express or implied, about the completeness, accuracy, or reliability of the information contained in this book. Note that the results of scientific and statistical research described in this book may be subject to change.

Editorial, design and indexing: Maria Carter
Production assistant: Hannah Phillips
Cover image: Master the Moment (India) on license from Shutterstock #1684775845

"If the misery of the poor be caused not by the laws of nature, but by our institutions, great is our sin."

CHARLES DARWIN

Contents

Contents

Introduction

The right nutrition at the right time is a mantra that is relevant throughout the lifetime of all individuals, but it is particularly potent during early life, when normal growth and development can provide the foundation for future health and wellbeing. There is increasing evidence that infant and young-child feeding is not only addressing the immediate nutritional needs of the child but also has a capability to nutritionally 'programme' the child for health and wellbeing in later life.

However, determining optimum nutrition in early life that will support current and future health is a challenge for scientists, health professionals, parents, policy-makers, governments and global health institutions. Moreover, infant feeding understandably attracts a range of special interest groups whose objective is to provide a civil society input and serve the needs of mothers and their partners. It is important that each of these stakeholders is willing to collaborate in the development of policies and practices that will lead to continuous improvement in nutritional care for the child and also provide reassurance to their family.

Yet for several decades the policy-making process has been a theatre of conflict with acrimony and division now deeply embedded between stakeholders. The key divisions are between the World Health Organization (WHO), industry, breastfeeding special interest groups, and more recently, health professionals who have been caught in the crossfire.

In 1981, the aim of the *International Code of Marketing of Breastmilk Substitutes* was:

> "... to contribute to the provision of safe and adequate nutrition for infants, by the protection and promotion of breastfeeding, and by ensuring the proper use of breastmilk substitutes, when these are necessary, on the basis of adequate information and through appropriate marketing and distribution".

This simple statement embraces two key aspects of infant feeding that remain fundamentally important today – the importance of protecting and promoting breastfeeding, and the acknowledgement that breastmilk substitutes may be necessary, but their proper use needs to be accompanied by appropriate marketing and promotion. As will become evident in this critique, fulfilment of this objective has not been achieved; instead there have been four decades of disharmony that continues to impact adversely on this incredibly important area of global public health.

There are several fundamental issues that continue to fuel this conflict.

- There are philosophical differences on the practice of infant feeding, ranging from idealism to realism. These conceptual differences are driving self-interest and division.

- There are inherent methodological complexities and ethical considerations that impact on breastfeeding research. Subsequently the evidence may not be sufficiently robust to prevent wide-ranging interpretation.

- With the conflict between stakeholders being allowed to endure

  for decades, acrimony and mistrust is now deeply embedded. This raises questions about effectiveness of leadership and strength of governance.

- Finally, and most concerning, is that this failure to deliver is set on a backdrop of the many millions of children worldwide who die each year before their fifth birthday. According to WHO 45% of these deaths are nutrition-related.

The thesis for this critique is that poor leadership and ineffective partnership-working are responsible for the failure to deliver infant and young-child feeding policies and practices that reflect the best scientific evidence, that meet the clinical needs of infants and young children worldwide, that are sensitive to the requirements of families living in the most diverse circumstances, and that are the product of due diligence conducted within a robust governance and regulatory structure.

The approach takes a health professional perspective to unpick the areas of conflict, appraise current policies and practices, reflect on the politics, and constructively attempt to find solutions that will make infant and young-child feeding policy more credible, desirable and achievable, and – most importantly – aim ultimately to save children's lives.

About the Author

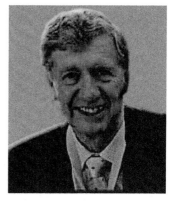

Professor Stewart Forsyth is Honorary Professor of Paediatrics, University of Dundee, and formerly Medical Director and Consultant Paediatrician, NHS Tayside, Scotland in the UK.

He graduated in medicine at the University of Glasgow in 1973, and after junior training posts in medicine, surgery and obstetrics and paediatrics, pursued a career in medical paediatrics specializing in neonatal intensive care in Edinburgh and Dundee and was appointed consultant paediatrician in 1983 with responsibility for the Neonatal Service in Dundee, Tayside. Subsequently he was appointed to Clinical Director roles and latterly was the Medical Director for the University Teaching Hospitals.

His Scotland-wide roles included Specialist Advisor on Medical Paediatrics to the Chief Medical Officer, Vice-Chair of the Scottish Governments Child Health Support Group, Chair of National Review of Neonatal Services in Scotland, and Deputy Convenor of Children in Scotland the largest children's charity in Scotland. More recently he has been Chair of the Early Nutrition and Later Health Task Force at the International Life Sciences Institute in Brussels. In 2012 he received the OBE award from HRH The Queen for contribution to children's health in Scotland.

He has had a longstanding research interest in infant and young-child nutrition and was the paediatric lead for the Dundee Infant Feeding Study which he initiated with his colleague Professor Peter Howie, Professor of Obstetrics and Gynaecology in 1986, and the results of the study were published in the *British Medical Journal* in 1990, 1993 and 1998. The study was one of the most comprehensive prospective assessments of the health benefits of breastfeeding during childhood in a developed country, and the published papers are still regularly referenced today. His most recent research has been related to the role of long chain polyunsaturated fatty acids in health and wellbeing in early life.

Professor Forsyth was commissioned to undertake advisory and health service reviews for the Scottish Government and also the UK Government, he is a past member of the Scottish Infant Feeding Advisory Group that was chaired by the Chief Nurse for Scotland, and in the past he has been a regular contributor to infant-feeding organizations including the Annual Conference of the Baby Friendly Initiative.

He is also Board Chairman of a Counselling organization based in Dundee and a founding member and former Chair of an organization called Parent-to-Parent which provides support for families with children with special needs.

Declaration of interests

In relation to research interests he has received grants from governments, national research funding organizations, charitable organizations and industry, and has received honoraria and expenses for presenting research findings at conferences in UK and abroad. Following his retirement from his clinical post he has undertaken consultancy work for DSM an international company that manufactures nutrient ingredients, and he specifically advises on fatty acids. DSM is not a breastmilk substitute manufacturer.

Author's publications relating to the content of this critique (in date order)

Howie PW, Forsyth JS, Ogston SA, *et al.* (1990) Protective effect of breastfeeding against infection. *British Medical Journal* 300, 11–16.

Forsyth JS, Ogston SA, Clark A, *et al.* (1993) Relation between early introduction of solid food to infants and their weight and illnesses during the first two years of life. *British Medical Journal* 306, 1572–76.

Wilson AC, Forsyth JS, Greene SA, *et al.* (1998) Relation of infant diet to childhood health: seven-year follow-up of a cohort of children in the Dundee infant feeding study. *British Medical Journal* 316, 21–25.

Forsyth S (2010) *International Code of Marketing of Breastmilk Substitutes* – three decades later time for hostilities to be replaced by effective national and international governance. *Archives of Disease in Childhood* 95, 769–70.

Forsyth S (2011) Policy and pragmatism in breastfeeding. *Archives of Disease in Childhood* 96: 909–10. DOI: 10.1136/adc.2011.215376.

Forsyth S (2012) FTSE, WHO Code and the infant-formula industry. *Annals of Nutrition and Metabolism* 60, 154–56. DOI: 10.1159/000337304.

Forsyth S (2013) Non-compliance with the *International Code of Marketing of Breastmilk Substitutes* is not confined to the infant-formula industry. *Journal of Public Health* 35, 185–90.

Forsyth S, Gautier S, Salem N Jr (2017) Dietary intakes of arachidonic acid and docosahexaenoic acid in early life – with a special focus on complementary feeding in developing countries. *Annals of Nutrition and Metabolism* **70**, 217–27.

Forsyth S (2018) Should the World Health Organization relax its policy of non-cooperation with the infant food industry? *Annals of Nutrition and Metabolism* 73, 160–62.

Forsyth S (2018) Is WHO creating unnecessary confusion over breastmilk substitutes? *Journal of Pediatric Gastroenterology and Nutrition* 67, 760–62.

Forsyth S (2018) Dietary docosahexaenoic acid and arachidonic acid in early life: what is the best evidence for policymakers? *Annals of Nutrition and Metabolism* 72, 210–22.

Forsyth S (2019) Formula milk studies couldn't exist without industry. *British Medical Journal* 364, l367.

Forsyth S (2019) What is opinion and what is evidence? *British Medical Journal* 366, l5395.

Forsyth S (2019) Infant feeding and conflict of interest: a healthcare perspective. *Annals of Nutrition and Metabolism* 75, 252–55. DOI: 10.1159/000504775).

Dattilo AM, Carvalho RS, Feferbaum R, Forsyth S, Zhao A (2020) Hidden realities of infant feeding: systematic review of qualitative findings from parents. *Behavioural Sciences (Basel)* 10, 83.

Forsyth S (2020) Should there be a comprehensive independent review of infant feeding policy-making? *Annals of Nutrition and Metabolism* 76, 201-206. DOI: 10.1159/000508455. Available at: https://www.karger.com/Article/FullText/508455/ (last accessed August 2022).

Forsyth S (2021) 40th anniversary of the international code of marketing of breastmilk substitutes. *The Lancet* 398, 1042.

Forsyth S (2022) Marketing of breast-milk substitutes revisited: new ideas for an old problem. *World Review of Nutrition and Dietetics* 124, 151-56. DOI: 10.1159/000516724.

Abbreviations and acronyms used in this book

AHRQ	Agency for Healthcare Research and Quality (US)
ANI	Access to Nutrition Index
ARA	arachidonic acid
BF	breastfeeding
BFHI	Baby-Friendly Hospital Initiative
BFI	Baby Friendly Initiative
BMI	body mass index
BMS	breastmilk substitute
BRCA	BReast CAncer (gene)
CCNFSDU	Codex Alimentarius Committee on Nutrition and Foods for Special Dietary Uses
CER	comparative effectiveness review
CFB	complementary foods and beverages
DHA	docosahexaenoic acid
DHS	demographic and health surveys
EBF	exclusive breastfeeding
ECOSOC	Economic and Social Council (UN)
EFSA	European Food Safety Authority
EGF	epidermal growth factor
EHC	Effective Health Care (programme)
EPA	eicosapentaenoic acid
ER	(o)estrogen receptors
ESG	environmental, social and governance
ESPGHAN	European Society for Paediatric Gastroenterology, Hepatology and Nutrition
ESPID	European Society for Paediatric Infectious Diseases

EAP	European Academy of Paediatrics
ESPNIC	European Society of Paediatric and Neonatal Intensive Care
ESPN	European Society for Paediatric Nephrology
ESPR	European Society for Paediatric Research
EUSEM	European Society of Emergency Medicine
EWG	Electronic Working Group, randomized controlled trials RCTs
FAO	Food Administration Organization
FSH	follicle-stimulating hormone
FT(SE)	Financial Times
GAIN	Global Alliance for Improved Nutrition
GI	gastrointestinal
GRACIF	Global Research Advisory Centre for Infant Feeding
GRADE	grading of recommendations assessment, development, and evaluation
hEGF	human epidermal growth factor
HER	hEGF receptors
IBFAN	International Baby Food Action Network
IGB	international governance board
IGBM	Interagency Group on Breastfeeding Monitoring
ILO	International Labour Organization
ILSI	International Life Sciences Institute
INFACT	Infant Feeding Action Coalition
ITT	intention-to-treat
LH	luteinizing hormone
MEP	Member of the European Parliament
MICS	multiple indicator cluster surveys
MMN	maternal multiple micronutrient
MoU	memorandum of understanding
NDA	nutrition, novel foods and food allergens
NGO	non-governmental organizations
NHS	National Health Service

NICE	National Institute for Health and Clinical Excellence
OECD	Organization for Economic Co-operation and Development
PR	progesterone receptors
PRLR	prolactin-related (genes)
PROBIT	Promotion of Breastfeeding Intervention Trial
PUFA	polyunsaturated fatty acids
RCPCH	Royal College of Paediatrics and Child Health
RR	relative risk
RUSFs	ready-to-use supplement foods
RUTFs	ready-to-use therapeutic foods
SAM	severe acute malnutrition
SDG	sustainable development goal
SGA	small for gestational age
SIDS	sudden infant death syndrome
STAG	scientific and technical advisory group
UN	United Nations
UNICEF	UN International Children's Emergency Fund
USAID	US Agency for International Development
WCRF	World Cancer Research Fund
WHA	World Health Assembly
WHO	World Health Organization

Illustrations

Boxes

3.1: Industry-related recommendations included in the International Code.

3.2: Healthcare-related recommendations included in the International Code.

3.3: Correspondence with the WHO Department of Nutrition for Health and Development (2010–2011).

3.4: Article from *BBC News Online* (July 2010): "*EXPERT CALLS FOR FORMULA-MILK WATCHDOG*".

3.5: Letter to Baby Milk Action (August 2010).

4.1: Mothers' attitudes to infant feeding—published letters (2020–2021).

5.1: Key statements from WHO in the consultation process of the EFSA paper.

5.2: Preventative nutritional interventions in children with acute malnutrition.

6.1: Summary of commentaries invited on *Journal of Public Health* article (2013).

7.1: The evolving 'clarification' of the term 'breastmilk substitutes'.

7.2: Confusion over breastmilk substitutes – breakfast options for a 2-year old child.

7.3: Invited commentary and subsequent correspondence in the *Journal of Pediatric Gastroenterology and Nutrition* (2018).

8.1: Potential interconnections between maternal breastfeeding and (a) childhood obesity and (b) maternal breast cancer.

8.2: Unpublished correspondence with Professor Michael Kramer of the PROBIT study (2014).

9.1: An evaluation framework for a pragmatic approach to nutrition policy issues in early life.

10.1: Personal correspondence with Professor Victora following publication of his article in *The Lancet Breastfeeding Series* (2016).

12.1: Extract from the Joint FAO/WHO Standards Programme Codex Committee on Nutrition and Foods for Special Dietary Uses (39th session, Berlin, Germany, 4–8 December 2017).

12.1: Industry involvement in policy-activist views.

14.1: Extracts from a letter from the Chief Executive of FTSE to the Chief Executive of Nestlé SA (November 2011).

Figures

Tables

CHAPTER 1

Three institutions

Global health governance is a highly contested landscape divided by conflicting ideas, interests, politics and economics,[1] and the area of global infant and young-child policymaking is no exception. Effective leadership and strategic direction at the highest level are critical success factors for all public and private organizations, whether they are global, national or local, and their performance will be enhanced by the qualities of vision, engagement and integrity. The principal institutions responsible for global infant and young child feeding policies are WHO, the United Nations (UN) and the Codex Alimentarius Commission.

The World Health Organization (WHO)

The WHO Constitution was adopted at an International Health Conference in New York on 22 July 1946 and took effect on 7 April 1948.[2] The opening paragraph of the WHO Constitution is:

"The States Parties to this Constitution declare, in conformity with the Charter of the United Nations, that the following principles are basic to the happiness, harmonious relations and security of all peoples".

Unfortunately, the words 'happiness' and 'harmonious' are not words that would be chosen today to describe the ambience of the process of delivering infant and young child feeding policies. This critically important area has been characterized by acrimony, division and mistrust, and why this dysfunctional behaviour has been allowed to continue for so long will be considered in this critique.

The WHO Constitution sets out the many responsibilities of the organization, which include:

- being the directing and coordinating authority in international health
- establishing and maintaining effective collaboration with the UN, specialized agencies, governmental health administrations, professional groups and other organizations as may be deemed appropriate
- to assist governments, upon request, in strengthening health services including maternal and child health.

An Interim Commission of WHO was formed in Geneva in 1946 to chart the roadmap for the future organization and oversee the draft of its constitution and other core documents. After establishing the WHO on 7 April 1948, the Interim Commission set a date of 24 June 1948 for convening the first Health Assembly in Geneva.

The purpose of the World Health Assembly (WHA) is to act as the governing body of the WHO. In 1948 the first WHA was attended by delegations from all but two of WHO's forty-eight member states. The WHA now includes a hundred and ninety-four member states. It is the world's highest health-policy setting body, composed of health ministers or their representatives from the member states, and a number of additional organizations with observer status. Its policy decisions are therefore subject to a wide range of geographical, political, economic and cultural perspectives, and this can impact both favourably and negatively on the effectiveness of the decision-making process.

The members of the WHA generally meet every year in May in Geneva at the Palace of Nations, the location of the WHO Headquarters. The main tasks of the WHA are to make decisions on major policy questions, to approve the WHO work programme and budget, and elect its Director-General.

A key committee within WHO and WHA structure is the Executive Board. The Board is the main link between the Secretariat of WHO and the WHA, with responsibilities that include acting as the executive organ of the Health Assembly and performing functions entrusted to it by the Health Assembly. The Secretariat comprises the Director-General and technical and administrative staff.

The principal departments within WHO with direct responsibilities for infant and young child feeding policy are the Department of Nutrition for Health and Development and the Department of Maternal, Newborn, Child and Adolescent Health.

WHO and the UN

The United Nations was founded on 24 October 1945 at the end of the Second World War, with the aims of:

- maintaining international peace and security
- developing friendly relations among nations on the basis of equality and the principle of self-determination
- fostering worldwide cooperation in solving economic, social, cultural and humanitarian problems.

There is a WHO office at the UN headquarters in New York, which provides the main contact with the UN system. The WHO office facilitates the participation of WHO and its Director-General in meetings of the UN Security Council, the General Assembly of the UN and the UN Economic and Social Council (ECOSOC), as well as other intergovernmental forums, interagency briefings, events and interaction with media including the UN Press Corps. A key objective of WHO's relationship with the UN system is to support the position of health in debates and decisions and to maintain the sustainable development agenda. Its most recent goals relate to the improvement of infant feeding and child nutrition and reducing stunting and child mortality by 2030.

The UN's International Children's Emergency Fund (UNICEF) was created by the UN in 1946 to provide food, clothing and healthcare to the children of post-World War II Europe. In 1953, UNICEF became a permanent part of the UN. At that time its name was shortened to United Nations Children Fund, but it is still referred to as UNICEF.[3]

UNICEF expanded the scope of its activities in the 1960s to include advocating for and advancing children's rights to education, healthcare and nutrition. In 1982, UNICEF commenced a new children's health programme that focused on monitoring growth, the use of oral rehydration therapy and the advocacy of breastfeeding and immunization. In 1989 the UN General Assembly adopted the Convention on the Rights of the Child, which UNICEF uses as guidance for its programmes.

UNICEF is governed by an Executive Board consisting of thirty-six members who are elected to terms of three years by the UN's Economic and Social Council. Each region that UNICEF serves is allocated a number of seats on the Executive Board, so all regions are represented. UNICEF is headquartered in New York and there are thirty-six national committees across the globe, which are non-governmental organizations (NGOs).

WHO and Codex Alimentarius

In May 1963, recognizing the importance of WHO's role in all health aspects of food, and considering its mandate to establish food standards, the 16th WHA approved the establishment of the Joint Food Administration Organization (FAO)/WHO Food Standards Programme, and adopted the statutes of the Codex Alimentarius Commission. The primary objectives of the Codex Alimentarius are to protect the health of consumers and to ensure fair practices are adopted within the food trade.[4] The Codex is not entirely independent of WHO, which provides administrative, managerial and financial support to the operation of the Codex Alimentarius Commission and its committees.

The Codex Alimentarius is a collection of international food standards that have been adopted by the Codex Alimentarius Commission. Its standards cover all the main foods, whether processed, semi-processed or raw. In infant and child health, it has developed standards for infant formula, follow-up formula and complementary foods. Its responsibilities also include the hygienic and nutritional quality of food, including microbiological norms, food additives, pesticide and veterinary drug residues, contaminants, labelling and presentation, and methods of sampling and risk analysis.

The main Codex Committee for infant and young-child nutrition is the Codex Committee on Nutrition and Foods for Special Dietary Uses (CCNFSDU), which has the remit of:

- studying specific nutritional problems assigned to it by the Commission
- advising the Commission on general nutrition issues
- drafting general provisions (as appropriate) concerning the nutritional aspects of all foods
- developing standards, guidelines or related texts for foods for special dietary uses in cooperation with other committees (where necessary)
- considering, amending (if necessary) and endorsing provisions on nutritional aspects proposed for inclusion in Codex standards, guidelines and related texts.

The current project of developing composition standards for infant formulas and follow-up formulas has been a long and tortuous process involving up to eight steps and taking as many years to complete. However, the group of organizations participating in the process is diverse, with government representatives from all countries together with a range of non-government organizations, industry representatives and professional and academic groups.

Performance of the three institutions

The performance of each of these institutions in directing optimum nutrition for infants and young children can be measured through outcomes for health and wellbeing – however, these are not encouraging. In 2020 it was reported that:

- the global mortality for children under five years of age is 4.9 million per year, of which 45% are nutrition related

- 149 million children under the age of five are suffering from the physical and cognitive effects of stunting
- 49 million are affected by wasting
- 40 million are overweight.[5]

Moreover, global breastfeeding rates remain disappointing and the global pandemic of childhood obesity is spreading.[6] More recently, in a series of articles in *The Lancet*, the gravity of the double burden of malnutrition[8]* was laid bare by the suggestion that previous interventions to improve nutrition and increase weight gain in malnourished infants and young children may have contributed to the increasing prevalence of children being both overweight and malnourished.[7]

Developing public health policies with the aim of ensuring that populations consume a healthy diet and maximize their potential for health and wellbeing can be complex. There are many nutritive and non-nutritive factors that can influence nutritional status; altering one or more of these factors may provide benefit, but because of the level of interdependence a change may also create a negative outcome. Failure to provide the right food at the right time to the right individuals has lifelong implications, and for this to be achieved decisions need to be made through the right procedures, with the right people with the right knowledge, and the process must be conducted in the right working environment.

With this backdrop, it is evident that infant and young-child feeding is not all about breastfeeding, although it tends to dominate policy and practice and is the driver of much of the debate around infant and young-child feeding. The focus needs to be on the provision of an integrated balanced diet that meets nutritional needs for all children within their individual living environment. This requires an inclusive approach to planning and delivery, which necessitates that all stakeholders have an opportunity to contribute their respective knowledge and skills.

The global institutions have a responsibility for establishing such a collective approach and they should not allow acrimony and division obstruct the development of the best nutrition solutions for infants and children. At all levels of the policy-making process, there should be evidence of engagement with consumers and effective partnership-working with all key stakeholders – and both should be underpinned by appropriate regulation and other governance systems.

The importance of effective engagement with the target population should never be underestimated. Failure to provide assurance that the process of policy development adheres to acceptable professional and governance standards negatively impacts on implementation and compliance. The key decision maker

---

*The double burden of malnutrition is characterised by the coexistence of undernutrition along with over-weightness and obesity.

in the global policy structure is the WHA, and this organization has responsibility for governing the WHO secretariat. However, it is unclear who governs the WHA. The decisions endorsed by the WHA can have an impact on every child and family worldwide, and thus to ensure these populations are adequately protected and supported, the decision-making process needs to be inclusive with input from all relevant stakeholders, and due diligence should be verified through externally agreed governance systems.

References

1. Lee K (2009) Understandings of global health governance: The contested landscape. In: Kay A, Williams OD (eds) *Global Health Governance: Crisis, Institutions and Political Economy*. Palgrave Macmillan. DOI: 10.1057/9780230249486_2.

2. WHO (2006) *Constitution of the World Health Organization. Basic Documents (45th edn) Supplement*. Available at: http://www.who.int/governance/eb/who_constitution_en.pdf (last accessed August 2022).

3. *UNICEF History*. Available at: https://www.unicef.org/history (last accessed August 2022).

4. *Codex Alimentarius International Food Standards*. Website homepage. Available at: https://www.fao.org/fao-who-codexalimentarius/en/ (last accessed August 2022).

5. UN (2019) *The Sustainable Development Goals Report 2019*. Available at: https://unstats.un.org/sdgs/report/2019/ (last accessed August 2022).

6. WHO (2014) *Report of the Commission on Ending Childhood Obesity. Implementation plan: Executive summary*. Available at: https://apps.who.int/iris/bitstream/handle/10665/259349/WHO–NMH–PND–ECHO–17.1–eng.pdf?sequence=1 (last accessed August 2022).

7. Branca F, Demaio A, Udomkesmalee E, *et al.* (2020) A new nutrition manifesto for a new nutrition reality. *The Lancet* 395, 8–10.

CHAPTER 2

Three policies

Optimum nutrition during infancy and early childhood is essential if children are to fulfil their growth, health and development potential. The 2019 UN report on sustainable goals reported that, although the mortality rate for children under five years is dropping, there are forty-nine million children worldwide under that age of five years who are 'wasted', with a very low body weight for height, and in contrast there are forty million who are overweight for height.[1] It is critically important that young-child feeding policies are sensitive to the nutritional requirements of children worldwide and respect the needs of children who may be living in sub-Saharan Africa and southern Asia or North America and Europe. To achieve this, policy-makers need to be receptive to the diversity of need and recognize that a 'one-size-fits-all' approach may be inappropriate. Moreover, it should be accepted that all key policymakers have a contribution to make to the policy-making process.

However, as stated previously, infant and young-child policymaking has a long and troubled history. Even today, the policymaking process is characterized by self-interest and division. The improvements in nutritional care that have led to increased survival and wellbeing of many children with acute and chronic disease were achieved by effective collaboration between scientists, clinicians and industry. However, in the critically important area of infant and young child nutrition, within the general population, infant feeding issues relating to policy and practice that were prominent four decades ago are still prevalent today.

The WHO and WHA, supported by the WHO Executive Board are responsible for developing and endorsing global policies on infant and young-child feeding. The process may involve a scientific and technical advisory group (STAG), a period of consultation, and working papers prepared by the WHO Secretariat that are then considered at the WHA. A decision to endorse the WHO recommendations is made by the WHA. The decisions are not legally binding, but all governments are 'urged' by the WHA to put them into effect.

There are three key global policies relating to infant and young-child feeding, namely 'the Code', the Innocenti Declaration and the WHO Global Strategy for infant and child feeding.

15

The Code

First is the *International Code of Marketing of Breastmilk Substitutes* (the Code).[2] On 23 May 1980, the Thirty-Third WHA supported the proposal that:

> *"… there should be an international code of marketing of infant formula and other products that are used as breastmilk substitutes".*

The WHA had previously expressed concern about declining breastfeeding rates and had recommended the following to the member states:

- to give priority to preventing malnutrition in infants and young children by supporting and promoting breastfeeding
- to take legislative and social action to facilitate breastfeeding
- to regulate the inappropriate promotion of infant foods that may be used to replace breastmilk.

WHO and UNICEF had previously responded to these concerns by convening a meeting in Geneva in October 1979. It was attended by a wide range of representatives including government officials, organizations of the UN system, NGOs and the infant-food industry. It was from that discussion that the concept of an *International Code of Marketing of Breastmilk Substitutes* emerged. It was subsequently presented to the WHA in May 1980. WHO and UNICEF were requested to take forward the preparation of the Code and were specifically asked to involve all concerned parties and reach a conclusion as soon as possible. The Fourth Draft of the Code was presented to the Executive Board, who agreed that it should be presented at the WHA in May 1981.

Dr Torbjørn Mork, Director-General of Health Services in Norway, and Vice-Chair of the Executive Board, delivered the Fourth Draft of the Code to the Thirty-fourth World Health Assembly. The text was unanimously adopted by the WHA as a minimum requirement to protect and promote appropriate feeding for infants and young children.[2] It was decided that the Code should be adopted as a *recommendation* (rather than a regulation) and that its implementation should be closely monitored according to existing WHO constitutional procedures, with progress assessed by future assemblies. The Code has not been updated since it was published in 1981, although the WHA has endorsed a number of subsequent resolutions.

Interestingly, the introductory comments by Dr Mork, which are appended as an Annex to the transcript of the Code, provide an insight into the original thinking, interpretation and purpose of the Code and specifically their views on what a 'breastmilk substitute' is, and what a 'complementary food' is, a subject that remains contentious four decades later. The debate continues because the definitions contained within the Code have allowed variation in interpretation and this is illustrated in Table 2.1.

Table 2.1: Excerpts from the introductory statement by the representative of the Executive Board to the 34th World Health Assembly on the subject of the draft International Code.

Statement from the Executive Board	Statement in the Code
'During the first 4–6 months of life, breastmilk alone is usually adequate to sustain the normal infant's nutritional requirements. Breastmilk may be replaced (substituted for) during this period by bona fide breastmilk substitutes, including infant formula. Any other food, such as cow's milk, fruit juices, cereals, vegetables, or any other fluid, solid or semisolid food intended for infants and given after this initial period, can no longer be considered as a replacement for breastmilk (or as its bona fide substitute). Such foods only complement breastmilk or breastmilk substitutes and are thus referred to in the draft code as complementary. They are also commonly called weaning foods or breastmilk supplement.' *Products other than bona fide breastmilk substitutes, including infant formula, are covered by the code only when they are 'marketed or otherwise represented to be suitable ... for use as a partial or total replacement of breastmilk.'*	*'The Code applies to the marketing, and practices related thereto, of the following products: breastmilk substitutes, including infant formula; other milk products, foods and beverages, including bottle fed complementary foods, when marketed or otherwise represented to be suitable, with or without modification, for use as a partial or total replacement of breastmilk.'* *For the purposes of this Code:* *'Breastmilk substitute means any food being marketed or otherwise presented as a partial or total replacement for breastmilk, whether or not suitable for that purpose'.* *'Complementary food means any food whether manufactured or locally prepared, suitable as a complement to breastmilk or to infant formula, when either become insufficient to satisfy the nutritional requirements of the infant. Such food is also commonly called 'weaning food' or 'breastmilk supplement'.*
Author comments	**Author comments**
This statement indicates the following: The WHO Executive Board referred to breast milk substitutes as the replacement or substitution of breastmilk during the first 4–6 months. • Any other fluids or foods given after this period are complementary foods. • Other than breastmilk substitutes, products are only covered by the Code when they are marketed or represented to be suitable as a partial or total replacement of breastmilk.	The lack of specificity in terms of time has allowed a diversity of interpretation that has generated debate and conflict for forty years. Questions remain, however, such as: • When is a breastmilk substitute no longer a breastmilk substitute? • When is a breastmilk substitute not a complementary food? • When is a complementary food no longer a complementary food? • When are milk and food products no longer within the scope of the Code?

This observation has relevance to more recent discussions about the definition of a breastmilk substitute and, in particular, when a breastmilk substitute is no longer considered to be a breastmilk substitute. In 2016, WHO officials, as a point of 'clarification', stated that all milk products marketed for children up to the age of three years should be understood to be breastmilk substitutes. It is difficult to align this interpretation with the comments of Dr Mork or the text of the Code document and this issue is discussed more fully in Chapter 7.

The Code clearly states that governments, NGOs, experts in various related disciplines, consumer groups and industry need to cooperate in activities aimed at improving maternal, infant and young-child health and nutrition. It was anticipated that the Code would provide the framework for this to be achieved, however the subsequent four decades have been the focus of continuing acrimony and division – and there are no signs of the hostilities resolving.[3] The infant formula industry is widely considered to be the *bête noire*, with frequent substantive claims that they adopt marketing and promotion practices that are not compliant with the Code; moreover, they are considered by WHO to be the underlying mechanism for the unfavourable static or decreasing breastfeeding rates across the developing and developed world. The response from WHO has been to place further restrictions on the marketing and promotion of infant formula through a series of additional resolutions.

Although the unprofessional marketing activities of the formula industry were the driving force for the introduction of the Code, the delivery of optimum nutrition to infants worldwide is a multi-stakeholder process, and systemic deficiency at any level may increase the risk of non-compliance with the Code. The Articles in the Code consider aspects of policy relating to governments, health services and parents, but there are no Articles specific for WHO, WHA and breastfeeding interest groups.

At the launch, the Code was viewed as a seminal policy, developed in partnership with all key stakeholders, including the infant-formula industry. It was agreed that the member states would communicate annually to the Director-General, providing information on any action taken to give effect to the principles and aim of the Code. In addition, the Director-General has to report in even-numbered years to the WHA on the status of implementation of the Code. It is also noted that (based on the conclusions of the status report) there should be proposals, if necessary, for revisions to the text of the Code and for measures required for its effective application.

An independent review of the Code not initiated by WHO (or WHA) noted in 2018 that:

"WHO and its partners must take active steps to ensure the Code can function as a coherent and clarified set of standards and provide better mechanisms for resolving difficulties in its interpretation and application. In particular, the Code's interaction with the use of commercial complementary foods must be guided by the broader objective of child nutrition and reflect the complexities of the relationship between breastfeeding and other nutrition imperatives".[4]

Further quotations from this important report are given in the *Addendum* to this chapter. Many of the identified issues relating to the Code are considered further in Chapter 3 and throughout this critique.

The Innocenti Declaration

The second major policy to be agreed was the Innocenti Declaration. This was done at the *Policymakers Meeting—Breastfeeding in the 1990s: A Global Initiative*, held at the Innocenti Centre in Florence on 30 July 1990.[5] The meeting included representation from thirty countries, of which only three were high-income. Organizational representation included UNICEF, WHO, the US Agency for International Development (USAID), the FAO and the World Bank. The co-sponsors of the meeting were USAID and the Swedish International Development Authority.

The output from this meeting, which has been called the *Innocenti Declaration on the Protection, Promotion and Support of Breastfeeding*, stated that all infants should be fed exclusively on breastmilk from birth to four to six months of age. Thereafter, children should continue to be breastfed, while receiving appropriate and adequate complementary foods, for up to two years of age or beyond.

There is an intriguing insight into how this recommendation emerged from one of the Swedish representatives,[6] who revealed that the arguments for the agreed recommendation were more anecdotal than scientific; evidence included the perception that children are more harmonious in later life if they are breastfed for five years or more. Reference was made to the Qur'an, which states that it is a child's right to be breastfed until the approximate age of two years. Finally, a Minister of Health from an African country questioned why his country should have sustained breastfeeding while other countries should not. However, it appears that the overriding concern was for children living in the most difficult circumstances that led to the Declaration.

Despite the lack of evidence in 1990 to underpin the recommendation of breastfeeding for two years or beyond for every child worldwide, this statement has been reaffirmed in all subsequent WHO global infant-feeding policy documents.

This is despite the evidence base for universality remaining weak, as reflected by a high level of non-compliance in families living in developed countries.

WHO Global Strategy for Infant and Young Child Feeding

In 2003, the WHO published a third policy document – the *Global Strategy for Infant and Young Child Feeding*.[7] They indicated that two key principles had guided this initiative: first, it should be grounded on the best available scientific and epidemiological evidence; second, it should be as participatory as possible. Their key global recommendation was that infants should be exclusively breastfed for the first six months of life to achieve optimal growth, development and health. Thereafter, to meet the child's evolving nutritional requirements, they should receive nutritionally adequate and safe complementary foods while breastfeeding continues for up to two years of age or beyond.

As part of the participatory process, the draft strategy was considered at country consultations in Brazil, China, the Philippines, Scotland, Sri Lanka, Thailand and Zimbabwe. WHO visited Scotland on 27 September 2000, where they received a consistent message from practitioners that there was strong support for the aspiration of improving the initiation and duration of exclusive breastfeeding, and the evidence base for developed countries supported a recommendation of exclusive breastfeed for four to six months.

It was assumed that Scotland had been chosen because of the Dundee Infant Feeding Study, conducted by our research team in the late 1980s and early 1990s. We reported associations between exclusive breastfeeding for three to four months with a reduction in gastrointestinal (and to a lesser extent respiratory) illness during infancy, and reduced childhood respiratory illness and lower blood pressure at the age of seven years.[8–10] The advice we gave to the WHO visitors, based on these findings, was that the policy should be led by the evidence. Several other large prospective studies supported this evidence. We recommended exclusive breastfeeding for four to six months, but also supported the view that in developed countries continuing breastfeeding should be for twelve months or beyond. We also warned that if targets are not realistic for individual countries, such as Scotland, the policy will have a negative impact.

In addition to the country consultations, there were six regional consultations comprising representatives from more than a hundred WHO national member states, as well as the participation of UNICEF, the FAO, the International Labour Organization (ILO), the International Lactation Consultant Association, the

International Baby Food Action Network (IBFAN), and the World Alliance for Breastfeeding Action. The organizations invited to this part of the consultation were enthusiastic breastfeeding advocates, so it is likely that the WHO were obtaining a highly selective viewpoint – one that some believe was favoured by WHO.

A review group was led by Professor Michael Kramer from McGill University in Montreal for a scientific perspective. His team had been very active in the area of infant feeding and health, and at that time had initiated the now renowned Promotion of Breastfeeding Intervention Trial (PROBIT) in Belarus (see Chapter 8). Professor Kramer and his colleague, Ritsuko Kakuma, were commissioned by WHO and the Cochrane Collaboration to undertake a systematic review of the optimal duration of exclusive breastfeeding. The initial results were published in 2002.[11] In their review, Kramer and Kakuma included sixteen independent studies that met the selection criteria; seven were from developing countries (two of which were controlled trials in Honduras) and nine of which were from developed countries and were all observational studies.

The review identified some weaknesses – both in the design and methodology – in many of these studies. For example, the two Honduran trials did not have high methodological quality ratings, yet they were considered to be superior to any of the observational studies. These observational studies were described as being of variable quality and their non-experimental designs were unable to exclude potential sources of confounding and selection bias. Further, the definitions of 'exclusive' breastfeeding varied considerably across the studies, leading to difficulties in separating *exclusive* breastfeeding from *predominant* breastfeeding.

Neither the trials nor the observational studies suggested that infants who continued to be exclusively breastfed for six months showed deficits in weight or length gain (although it was noted that larger sample sizes were required). It was also reported that the data were extremely limited with respect to iron status. It was also suggested that – at least in developing country settings where newborn iron stores may be suboptimal – exclusive breastfeeding without iron supplementation for six months may compromise haematological status. The authors of the review reported on their own observational analysis of a large, randomized trial (in Belarus) that gastrointestinal infection was recorded in 7.4% of infants receiving three months exclusive breastfeeding compared to 5.0% of infants exclusively fed for six months.[11] However, there was no difference in hospital admissions.

Despite the obvious concerns regarding the quality of the data, the review concluded that the available evidence demonstrated no apparent risks in recommending, as public health policy, exclusive breastfeeding for the first six months of life in both developing *and* developed country settings. However, they weren't able to make a statement indicating that there were significant additional health benefits from six months' exclusive breastfeeding compared to four months. Kramer and colleagues subsequently followed up the Belarus cohort, when the children were 6.5, 11.5 and 16 years. This is discussed in more detail in Chapter 8.

The WHO invited a group of experts to review Kramer and Kakuma's systematic review, to formulate recommendations for practice on the optimal duration of exclusive breastfeeding, and to provide recommendations for research needs in this area.[12] Because the Expert Consultation considered there were some deficiencies in the review, they included published studies that didn't meet the selection criteria for the review. In particular, no mortality data were available that directly compared exclusive breastfeeding for four to six months versus six months.

After considering the modified data set, the Expert Consultation concluded that exclusive breastfeeding should be for six months, with the introduction of complementary foods and continued breastfeeding thereafter, but they did identify a number of caveats that are considered in more detail in Chapter 4. They made the point that this recommendation applied to all populations and acknowledged that some mothers would be unable to (or choose not to) follow the advice, so should be supported to optimize their infants' nutrition.

The Expert Consultation also recognized the importance of complementary feeding at six months of age and recommended the introduction of nutritionally adequate, safe and appropriate complementary foods – in conjunction with continued breastfeeding. The *Global Strategy for Infant and Young Child Feeding*, which included six months exclusive breastfeeding and continuing breastfeeding for two years and beyond, was endorsed by the WHA in May 2002 and published in 2003.

It is important to reflect on the 'back story' of the policy of infant and young child feeding and be reminded of the knowns and unknowns that underpinned the thinking at the time. It is also important to consider whether, some twenty years later, this advice is still relevant and meets the needs of children across the world. This is considered further in Chapter 4 and at different points throughout this book.

Conclusion

The three pillars of global policy on infant and young-child feeding have been in place for several decades. It was initially anticipated that they would provide the foundation for global improvements in infant and young nutrition, based on sound science, policy and practice. Revisiting the origins of these policies is an illuminating exercise, and it provides a reminder that, at that time, the policies were predominantly based on subjective reasoning and some wishful thinking – *rather* than solid evidence. For many involved in infant-feeding practice today there is a belief that this philosophical rather than evidential approach continues to prevail.

Viewing the three policies retrospectively, especially with a lens that stretches back twenty to forty years, the evidence clearly indicates that all three policies have significant gaps between their original aspirations and later achievements. And each one has been the source of uncertainty and division within the infant feeding community. It is therefore important that these polices should not be perceived as inscribed in tablets of stone, and in the interests of future engagement and commitment, there must be discussion on their utility and value, within the context of the need for sensitivity to the diversity of societal change.

Addendum

Reference is made in this chapter to the first independent review of the Code, which was undertaken by Angela Evans in a report entitled *Food for Thought*. Angela Evans is a distinguished lawyer based in Stockholm, Sweden, who specializes in international law and human rights. She has a broad international practice with a particular focus on business and human rights. Her report was initially commissioned by the UN Secretary-General's Special Envoy for Health and was completed under the auspices of the Breastfeeding Innovations Team. The Breastfeeding Innovations Team is a global network of more than two hundred and fifty individuals and organizations that are committed to accelerating the development and adoption of innovations that have the greatest potential to increase access to breastmilk for babies – especially the most vulnerable.

The content of Evans' report is encapsulated here through a selection of quotations that were highlighted within the report by Evans herself:

> *"For a document with such an important objective, the Code is shrouded in an unacceptable degree of uncertainty and controversy."*

> *"There are well-founded concerns amongst stakeholders that the ambiguity and acrimony surrounding the Code is having negative side effects not only on the promotion of breastfeeding, but on broader efforts to promote any kind of responsible role for the private sector in child nutrition."*

> *"It is difficult to follow the rules when it is challenging to find out what the rules are."*

"… champions of infant and child health must persevere to establish better collective insight into how Code implementation impacts marketing practices and infant feeding in today's world. This is essential in order to understand what future action can and should look like."

"Industry and its civil society stakeholders have persistently diverged in their interpretation of the Code."

"Currently, however, there is no sufficiently authoritative, impartial, and trusted mechanism(s) for establishing compliance."

"A carefully architected and publicized dialogue between UN and industry at the most senior level could provide the right kind of publicity and accountability that industry conduct needs in order to be pressed to reform."

"Without better mechanisms for dialogue, monitoring and trust development, the historical toxicity surrounding the marketing of breastmilk substitutes will likely continue to infect broader efforts to engage the private sector as a partner for nutrition."

References

1. UN (2019) *The Sustainable Development Goals Report 2019*. Available at: https://unstats.un.org/sdgs/report/2019/ (last accessed August 2022).

2. WHO (1981) *International Code of Marketing of Breastmilk Substitutes*. Geneva, WHO. ISBN 92-4-154160-1. Available at: http://apps.who.int/iris/bitstream/handle/10665/40382/9241541601.pdf?sequence=1 (last accessed September 2022).

3. Forsyth JS (2010) International Code of Marketing of Breastmilk Substitutes – three decades later time for hostilities to be replaced by effective national and international governance. *Archives of Diseases of Childhood* 95, 769–70.

4. Evans A (2018) *Food for thought. An independent assessment of the International Code of Marketing of Breastmilk Substitutes*. Breastfeeding Innovation Team. Available at: https://medium.com/@JustACTIONS/food-for-thought-an-independent-assessment-of-the-international-code-of-marketing-of-breast-milk-1d8d704ee612 (last accessed August 2022).

5. *Innocenti declaration on the protection, promotion and support of breast-feeding* (1990). Available at: https://worldbreastfeedingweek.org/2018/wp-content/uploads/2018/07/1990-Innocenti-Declaration.pdf (last accessed August 2022).

6. Greiner T (2000) *The history and importance of the Innocenti Declaration*. Available at: http://arnone.de.unifi.it/mami/congresso/greiner.pdf (last accessed August 2022).

7. WHO/UNICEF (2003) *Global strategy for infant and young-child feeding.* Available at: http://apps.who.int/iris/bitstream/10665/42590/1/9241562218.pdf?ua=1&ua=1 (last accessed March 2022).

8. Howie PW, Forsyth JS, Ogston SA, *et al.* (1990) Protective effect of breastfeeding against infection. *British Medical Journal* 300, 11–16.

9. Forsyth JS, Ogston SA, Clark A, *et al.* (1993) Relation between early introduction of solid food to infants and their weight and illnesses during the first two years of life. *British Medical Journal* 306, 1572–76.

10. Wilson AC, Forsyth JS, Greene SA, *et al.* (1998) Relation of infant diet to childhood health: seven-year follow-up of a cohort of children in the Dundee infant feeding study. *British Medical Journal* 316, 21–25.

11. Kramer MS, Kakuma R (2002) Optimal duration of exclusive breastfeeding. *Cochrane Database of Systematic Reviews* 20128, CD003517. DOI: 10.1002/14651858.CD003517. PMID: 11869667. Available at: https://pubmed. ncbi.nlm.nih.gov/11869667/ (last accessed February 2022).

12. WHO (2021) *The optimal duration of exclusive breastfeeding. Report of an expert consultation.* Available at: https://apps.who.int/iris/bitstream/handle/10665/67219/WHO_NHD_01.09.pdf?ua=1 (last accessed February 2022).

CHAPTER 3

Why has the Code been associated with decades of conflict?

The Code is underpinned by eleven articles, and of these:

ARTICLE 1 sets out the aim of the Code, which is to contribute to the provision of safe and adequate nutrition for infants, by the protection and promotion of breastfeeding and by ensuring the proper use of breastmilk substitutes. In particular, the aim emphasizes the need for milk substitutes to be based on adequate information and to be provided through appropriate marketing and distribution.[1]

ARTICLES 2 and **3** cover the scope and definitions used in the Code. Subsequent articles relate to government responsibility for ensuring that objective and consistent information is provided on infant and young-child feeding for use by families and those involved in the field of infant and young-child nutrition. There are recommendations for manufacturers and distributors of breastmilk substitutes, with specific reference to advertising and labelling, and advice and information for healthcare systems and healthcare workers that focuses on the encouragement of breastfeeding and promotion of the principles of the Code.

ARTICLE 10 provides recommendations on the quality and standards for milk substitutes.

ARTICLE 11 sets out arrangements for monitoring the implementation of the Code.

The introduction to the Code clearly states that governments, organizations of the UN system, NGOs, and experts in various related disciplines, consumer groups and industry need to cooperate in activities that are aimed at improving maternal, infant and young-child health and nutrition. However, the evidence from the last four decades indicates that the aspiration of collective cooperation has not been fulfilled. There has been an unrelenting series of disputes, predominantly relating to alleged violations of the Code, which have provoked high-profile acrimonious exchanges, boycotts and legal proceedings.[2]

An internet search of the Code is dominated by claims of violation raised by NGOs (predominantly IBFAN and Baby Milk Action) against milk-formula companies, predominantly Nestlé. Most striking is the absence of a website commissioned by an official independent governance body that provides comprehensive and validated data on such claims of violation and their outcomes.

The arrangements for implementation and monitoring of the Code are set out in Article 11. They state that individual governments should take action to give effect to the principles and aim of the Code and, if appropriate, consider the adoption of national legislation, regulations or other suitable measures. Governments are also advised that they can seek the cooperation of the WHO, UNICEF and other agencies of the UN system. Article 11 also emphasizes that manufacturers and distributors of products within the scope of the Code should – independently of any other measures taken for implementation of this Code – regard themselves as responsible for monitoring their marketing practices according to the principles and aim of the Code, and for taking steps to ensure that their conduct at every level conforms to them.

The Code also states that NGOs, professional groups, institutions and individuals should have the responsibility of drawing the attention of manufacturers and distributors to activities that are incompatible with the principles and aim of the Code (so that appropriate action can be taken) and that the appropriate governmental authority should also be informed.

The recommendations contained within the Code have been classified as relevant to industry or health[3] and are shown in Boxes 3.1 and 3.2. It is noted that the recommendations are aimed at the practice of industry, healthcare and indirectly parents, and there are no recommendations specifically relating to the practice of WHO, WHA or activist groups.

Unfortunately, the evidence indicates that this rather complex multi-agency monitoring framework has failed to deliver effective corporate governance. It is probably not surprising that each of the components of this self-regulatory structure continue to manifest aspects of self-interest, which is likely to continue in the absence of an 'ombudsman' or an independent body with the authority to arbitrate and ensure that actions taken by respective parties are in keeping with the spirit of the Code.

In the absence of effective governance and validated information from an official international or national regulatory body, a number of self-appointed monitoring groups have opportunistically filled this vacuum. The most influential of these is

**Box 3.1: Industry-related recommendations included in
the International Code[3]**

- There should be no advertising or other forms of promotion of the products.
- Manufacturers or distributors should not provide free product samples to mothers.
- Manufacturers or distributors should not distribute any gifts or articles to mothers.
- Marketing personnel should not seek direct or indirect contact with mothers. Labels should provide the necessary information about a product.
- Labels should state the superiority of breastfeeding and provide information on appropriate preparation of a product.
- Labels or the container should not have any picture or text that idealizes the use of infant formula.
- Labels should indicate the ingredients used, the composition, storage conditions required, batch number and date by which the product is to be consumed.

**Box 3.2: Healthcare-related recommendations included in
the International Code[3]**

- Facilities of the healthcare system should not be used for display of products.
- No healthcare services should use professional service representatives provided or paid by manufacturers or distributors.
- Health workers should encourage and protect breastfeeding.
- Health professionals should be provided with scientific and factual information about the product.
- No information to health workers should imply or create a belief that bottle feeding is superior to breastfeeding.
- No material or financial inducements to promote products should be offered to health workers or members of their families.
- Health workers should not give samples of infant formula to mothers members of their families.

IBFAN. The Code does encourage NGOs to draw the attention of manufacturers and distributors to activities that are incompatible with the principles and aim of the Code, however it is clear that it is difficult for these organizations to access all relevant information and provide an independent and fully informed view. Moreover, from the way that they are constituted, and the methods that they have adopted, it is unlikely they will be able to embrace the confidence of all relevant parties.

Within individual countries there is a need for governments to provide a more transparent governance structure that has clearly defined responsibilities for ensuring there are reliable and sustainable systems in place to underpin the effective delivery of the Code. The remit of such a national governing body could be:

- to oversee the process for responding to claims of violation
- to ensure that standards are being met for the investigation of claims of violation, and
- to make relevant information available in the public domain for example, a register of all claims of violation (with the outcome and action taken).

For this to be achieved, it would be a priority to review all of the relevant Code monitoring processes and to take measures to make sure that reliable and sustainable systems are in place. Robust data will be required to provide assurance to the relevant parties, to determine more clearly the extent of the issue, and to advise on appropriate actions. This group could also have broader governance responsibilities relating to the implementation of the Code. It is essential for the membership of such a body to have the confidence of *all* interested parties, and therefore its members will need a range of skills and expertise that assure governments, industry, NGOs, professional groups, institutions and individuals that they are informed, transparent and independent.

In addition to strengthening the governance arrangements at a national level, it is also important to have reliable systems in place that demonstrate effective international accountability. Although international monitoring systems have been developed, the current arrangements dictate that it is the responsibility of individual WHO member states to decide what actions, if any, are taken in response to a claim of violation of the Code. There is a risk that there may be global inconsistency in approach and outcome. One potential scenario is that a non-governmental organization from one country claims that a violation took place in another country, and the milk-formula company that is allegedly responsible is based in yet another country. Violation claims that cross national and continental boundaries should be addressed within a framework of international governance that is transparent, consistent and sustainable. This issue is discussed in more detail in Chapter 14.

In the previously mentioned excellent independent review by Angela Evans,[4] it was concluded:

> *"For a document with such an important objective, the Code is shrouded in an unacceptable degree of uncertainty and controversy. The national transposition of the Code into domestic laws has been patchy and inconsistent. Corporate adherence to the Code is hotly contested amongst stakeholders and there is a lack of trusted and transparent systems for ensuring stakeholder accountability".[4]*

This report provided a series of recommendations relating to Code provisions, implementation and corporate conduct. It is also important to consider these findings within the broader aspects of policymaking for infant and young-child feeding, and thus contribute to a more holistic approach to the improvement of nutritional health and wellbeing of children worldwide.

The Code – is it time for a new perspective?

It is evident that, since it was launched in 1981, the Code has had a 'bumpy ride' and is still at the centre of controversy relating to infant nutrition. As described, measures have been taken to try and legitimize it, but uncertainties remain. A central issue is that WHO have taken the view that stakeholders should not have a professional working relationship with the infant food industry. Unfortunately, WHO took the line (and still do) that health professionals could be influenced by the salesmanship of industry personnel, and therefore such contact should be considered as a potential conflict of interest, because it may negatively impact on breastfeeding. Clearly, for WHO to make such allegations, unequivocal evidence of misconduct or criminality needs to be presented by the policymakers, and no such evidence has been formally produced. At a practical level, a key question is: After forty years, what has the disengagement of stakeholders from industry achieved? The answer is not encouraging. Breastfeeding rates are disappointing, and Nestlé is now the largest food and beverage company in the world.

A key aspect of conflict resolution is effective communication between the conflicting parties. On that evidence, an alternative approach to the Code strategy could be to *increase* communication between stakeholders and industry.

The basis for this approach would be that the different stakeholders will be able to apply their respective knowledge and expertise to hold industry to account and through a constructive and informative exchange a collective sense of direction should be achieved. This should include agreement on the boundaries of industry involvement in policymaking and also the delivery of service. If relations between the stakeholders, including industry, had been normal (that is, treating each other with trust and respect, sharing information, and making collective decisions), could there have been a more timely and effective response to the child obesity pandemic?

Finally, can industry assure stakeholders that they will respond responsibly to such an opportunity? The answer is that we need to find out. Forty years has been long enough to learn that stakeholder disengagement from industry does *not* work and may have serious consequences. A key element of best practice is to ensure that there is effective engagement between all partners, and this should be viewed as an essential governance standard.

Conclusion

The Code is a seminal document, but to maintain this status it needs to remain relevant to contemporary society. If it does not, there is a risk that it presents as a problem, rather than a solution. The reluctance of WHO/WHA to initiate a formal review of the Code after forty years raises the suspicion that they are concerned the Code (in its current form) would not survive close examination. The current practice of 'clarifying' aspects of the Code through random 'subsequent resolutions', which are proposed by WHO and agreed by WHA, lacks credibility, as they do not command the same extensive attention and consultation that a revised Code would attract.

Moreover, observers who are more sceptical may perceive this as a tactic by WHO officials to change meaning of the Code without going down the path of an extensive review. The credibility of this bureaucratic balancing act may be acceptable for minor adaptations relating to the Code, but when applied to something as fundamental as the definition of a breastmilk substitute – a term included in the title of the Code document – it is not surprising that questions are being asked on matters of transparency, due diligence and integrity. For the Code to feel relevant to the other stakeholders, the 'clarifications' and 'subsequent resolutions' should reflect the broader collective approach that underpinned the original development of the Code, whereas at present WHO and breastfeeding activist colleagues appear to consider this as their prerogative and consequently, their input has begun to alter meaning and the spirit of the Code and if this continues the sense of ownership and commitment to the Code by the wider stakeholder community will further decline.

Issues relating to the Code are increasingly permeating through many aspects of infant and young-child policymaking, and at some point – preferably soon – officials will need to face the prospect of a review of the Code. For such an important aspect of global public health, a more coherent and contemporary set of infant feeding standards is required if twenty-first-century governance standards are to be met. Furthermore, a review may reveal that under the blanket of acrimony and division there is actually a large area of common ground within the Code, and most of the issues relate to interpretation or, to be more accurate, misinterpretation.

Addendum I

This chapter is based on a previously published article: Forsyth S (2010) *International Code of Marketing of Breastmilk Substitutes* – three decades later time for hostilities to be replaced by effective national and international governance *Archives of Diseases in Childhood* 95, 769–70.

I attempted to engage with WHO to raise some of the issues within the article. As the 30th anniversary of the Code was about to take place I wondered if it was timely to review the Code. I had an initial telephone conversation with one of the Team at WHO's Department of Nutrition for Health and Development regarding the paper and was asked to send a copy to them. I was told they would discuss it and come back to me, but no response was received. The content of the emails is shown in Box 3.3 over the following pages.

Box 3.3: Correspondence with the WHO Department of Nutrition for Health and Development (2010–2011)

First email (4 September 2010)

I attach a copy of my paper which was published online by the Archives of Disease in Childhood in July, and it will be in the October edition of the journal.

You will see that I particularly highlight the continuing hostilities between breastfeeding support groups and infant-formula companies, especially Nestlé. I believe that this continuing conflict is not only contrary to the spirit of the Code, which specifically encourages cooperation between the key parties, but continues to seriously undermine effective implementation of the Code. As long as this policy continues to be overshadowed by campaigns, boycotts and legal actions, it will not deliver the global health benefits that were anticipated when it was launched three decades ago.

You will see that I believe that there is a need for more effective governance of the Code at both national and international levels and an important outcome of this process would be the publication of robust data on the investigation and outcome of claims of violation. Without official data on claims of violation it is difficult for the general public and health professionals to make an informed judgement on compliance with the Code.

I think it is important that there is an acknowledgement of the 30th anniversary of the publication of the Code and this can provide an opportunity to review progress over the last thirty years, to address current issues and to consider future goals. There has been considerable interest in my paper, and I believe that a high-level event during 2011 would be welcomed by all key parties.

Second email (5 October 2010)

I write to inform you that my paper relating to the WHO Code is now published in hard copy in the current edition of *Archives of Disease in Childhood* and I believe that it is likely to generate some correspondence that will be published shortly. As I indicated previously I would appreciate any comments from the WHO Code team.

"From the email exchange that I have received, there is a desire to acknowledge the thirty-year anniversary of the Code and to take the opportunity to celebrate what has been achieved, address current issues, and consider future goals. Clearly it would be important for WHO to take a leading role on this proposal and I would welcome your thoughts.

Third email (3 February 2011)

I attach a copy of an email I sent in September last year when I was interested to know if WHO had plans to acknowledge the 30th anniversary of the publication of the Code. Following my paper, which I sent previously, a number of professional and related colleagues have indicated that this would be an appropriate time to review progress of implementation of the Code and an opportunity to consider ongoing issues. I wondered if you are able to respond to this email and if not, is there someone else that I should be contacting.

Fourth letter to Department of Nutrition for Health and Development (3 February 2011)

In the absence of a response from Dr S the email was sent to Dr C. No response was received.

Addendum II

When the original article was published in the *Archives of Disease in Childhood* there was considerable media interest, including an article on *BBC News Online* (Box 3.4).

Box 3:4: Article from *BBC News Online* (27 July 2010)

EXPERT CALLS FOR FORMULA-MILK WATCHDOG

A Scots expert has said disputes over the use of formula milk have hampered improvements in child nutrition. Professor Stewart Forsyth called for an ombudsman to oversee the voluntary Code on how the milk is marketed, nearly thirty years after it was established. He said a multi-agency approach to monitoring the Code was not working, because the self-regulatory structure resulted in claim and counterclaim. Mistrust has now developed between key agencies, he wrote in a health journal.

The article is published in the *Archives of Disease in Childhood*, a specialist title produced by the *British Medical Journal* (BMJ). The Code, which was established in 1981 and is monitored by the World Health Organization, contains eleven articles covering marketing and distribution, quality standards and government responsibilities. However, Prof. Forsyth, formerly of NHS Tayside, said the Code – which was intended to foster global cooperation between governments, industry and aid agencies – had instead been mired in three decades of often bitter dispute.

It is probably not surprising that each of the components of this self-regulatory structure continue to manifest aspects of self-interest, and this is likely to continue in the absence of an 'ombudsman' or independent body with the authority to arbitrate and ensure that actions taken by respective parties are in keeping with the spirit of the code.

Addendum III

There was a response from the Policy Director of Baby Milk Action on 30 July 2010, who was very concerned about the implication within my article that Baby Milk Action is keeping 'hostilities' going to the detriment of infant health. It was noted that this inference had been picked up in several media articles and referred to a statement that the thirty-year-old Code "*is mired by a series of alleged violations and boycotts, which are counterproductive to the Code's goal'*. They were concerned that I failed to mention that Baby Milk Action, and their many partners have been working successfully over decades for effective implementation of the Code and subsequent relevant Resolutions of the WHA, and that these have been introduced in legislation in over sixty countries, where these laws are monitored and enforced, and having a significant impact. They acknowledged the need for a governance body to be independent, but wanted clarification on what this means, how this would work, and whether it would monitor the current UK legislation or the full Code (which are very different things). They also noted that they had asked Nestlé many times to set out its terms and conditions for an independent expert tribunal to investigate claim and counter claim, but this had not been forthcoming. I wrote a response (Box 3.5) to Baby Milk Action but did not receive a reply.

Box 3.5: Letter to Baby Milk Action (2 August 2010)

Thank you for your email and I am happy to respond to your concerns.

Can I begin by saying that I fully appreciate that Baby Milk Action and its related organizations have made significant global achievements in relation to implementation of the Code and in enabling improvements in breastfeeding practice worldwide. I do believe, however, that you may have been more successful if it had been possible for your activities to have been in close partnership with the other key parties, especially the formula industry. I appreciate that your dealings with the milk-formula companies have been frustrating and this has triggered the various campaigns and boycotts. However, it is for that reason that I state in my paper that there is a need for formal governance measures to be in place that will have the necessary authority to ensure the companies and any other relevant parties cooperate with the implementation and delivery of the Code.

In response to your question, I strongly believe that the governance arrangements should apply to all articles in the Code and, therefore, this has significant relevance for healthcare workers and healthcare systems, as well as formula companies.

Although you clearly felt that my paper was critical of your organization, my primary focus was on the UK Government and its failure to provide evidence of robust and effective monitoring of the Code. I was not intending to be

---

critical when I said that Baby Milk Action had self-appointed and had been opportunistic but was merely highlighting that you had filled the governance vacuum and opportunistically initiated various monitoring systems.

As an early action following the publication of my paper, I am keen to encourage a meeting with government officials to consider the governance arrangements for the Code in the UK and how these can be 'scaled up' to meet our respective needs. For this meeting to have authority and impact, participants should include representatives from health, Baby Milk Action and the formula industry. The objective of the meeting would be to encourage the government to recognize the importance of an independent, transparent and informed governance system and to consider what action needs to be taken to enable that to happen.

From my perspective we will need to convince them that this will have the support of the key parties and we would be willing to participate. Would you be willing to support this approach?

I look forward to your thoughts on the above. I am happy to discuss and if there is sufficient common ground I would be pleased to meet to discuss in more detail.

References

1. WHO (1981) International Code of Marketing of Breastmilk Substitutes. Available at: https://apps.who.int/iris/bitstream/handle/10665/40382/9241541601.pdf?sequence=1&isAllowed=y (last accessed February 2022).

2. Forsyth S (2010) International Code of Marketing of Breastmilk Substitutes – three decades later time for hostilities to be replaced by effective national and international governance. *Archives of Diseases in Childhood* 95, 769–70.

3. Forsyth S (2021) Marketing of breastmilk substitutes revisited: new ideas for an old problem. World Review of Nutrition and Dietetics 124, 1–6. DOI: 10.1159/000516724.

4. Evans A (2018) Evans A (2018) *Food for thought. An independent assessment of the International Code of Marketing of Breastmilk Substitutes. Breastfeeding Innovation Team.* Available at: https://medium.com/@JustACTIONS/food-for-thought-an-independent-assessment-of-the-international-code-of-marketing-of-breast-milk-1d8d704ee612 (last accessed April 2022).

CHAPTER 4

Why have breastfeeding policies failed to engage with populations?

In early life, infants and young children require a continuum of optimal nutrition to meet their energy and nutrient requirements. The key food sources during this period are breastmilk, infant formula (if required) and complementary foods. It is important for infant-feeding policy to set out the need for a balanced diet, highlighting the importance of the interdependence of breastmilk and complementary foods to achieve normal growth and development, and recognizing that this nutritional balance may be influenced by both nutritive and non-nutritive factors.

For policy to be effective, it needs to constructively engage with the target populations. For infant-feeding policy, the key populations are parents and their health professionals, who must have a common understanding of what is being proposed and believe that the policy will serve the needs of children. If this is not achieved, parents will not experience a sense of trust and ownership of the policy, which can lead to disengagement. There is conclusive evidence to indicate that infants should be breastfed and that they need to be introduced to nutritious complementary foods, with progress towards a balanced family diet. So there is a large area of common ground, and when you analyze what it is that causes so much acrimony and division it predominantly distils down to the timing of these dietary transitions.

It is argued that the difficulties are not related to the *actual* commodities – that is, breastmilk, infant formula (if required) or complementary foods – but to the structures and rules that have been placed, layer upon layer, on the basic infant-feeding model. It needs to be understood that forty years of acrimony, division, conflict, boycotts and legal proceedings are not the result of parents, or any of the other stakeholders, not wishing to support breastfeeding; rather, it is the nature of the recommendations, resolutions and threats of legislation and sanctions that have been put in place to enforce specified timings of the nutritional transitions, when the evidential justification is considered by many as not good enough.

Exclusive breastfeeding

The optimum duration of exclusive breastfeeding is a subject of continuing debate. In 2010, Fewtrell and colleagues[1] challenged the evidence underpinning the 2002 WHA endorsement of the recommendation that in both developing and developed countries exclusive breastfeeding should be carried out for a minimum of six months. They questioned whether there was sufficient evidence to support the change from four to six months in developed countries, and they also suggested that the six-month policy could be disadvantageous to some infants. The hostility towards the academics for raising the question was considerable, and the WHO reaffirmed their view that all mothers worldwide should exclusively breastfeed for six months and continue breastfeeding for two years or beyond.[2]

In considering the optimum period for exclusive breastfeeding, it is important to give due consideration to related nutritive and non-nutritive influencing factors. There is strong scientific and clinical consensus that for developing countries the optimal duration of exclusive breastfeeding should be six months. This relates to the dangers of poor hygiene, the lack of clean water and sanitation, and the possible inadequate supply of nutritious complementary foods.

However, much of the debate in developed countries has centred on the micronutrient adequacy of six months of exclusive breastfeeding, the supportive evidence for complementary foods to be introduced between four and six months, and uncertainty regarding the magnitude of the additional health benefits from six months of exclusive breastfeeding compared to four to six months in high-income settings.

For developed countries in the early 1990s there was a general consensus across scientists, clinicians, policy-makers and members of the general public that exclusive breastfeeding for a minimum period of four months (with complementary foods introduced after four months and before six completed months) offered significant health benefits in infancy and early childhood. More recent studies have confirmed that these feeding recommendations *do* provide health benefits to infants and young children in developed countries, but the WHO – strongly supported by breastfeeding interest groups – chose to recommend exclusive breastfeeding for six months. Over the last twenty years there has been a considerable effort to find unequivocal evidence in support of this decision.

As previously mentioned, the initial Cochrane systematic review of the optimal duration of exclusive breastfeeding (funded by WHO) was undertaken by Kramer and Kakuma and initially published in 2002,[3] with subsequent updates, the most recent being in 2012.[4] They concluded that infants who are exclusively breastfed for six months experience less morbidity from gastrointestinal infection than those who are exclusively breastfed for three months. The latest Cochrane report in 2012[4] stated that exclusive breastfeeding (for six months versus three to four months, with continued mixed breastfeeding thereafter) reduces gastrointestinal infection and helps mothers lose weight and prevent pregnancy, but it has no long-term impact on allergic disease, growth, obesity, cognitive ability or behaviour.

It seems clear that the decision on six months of exclusive breastfeeding was strongly influenced by the data on gastrointestinal illness. In the Belarus study undertaken by Kramer and Kakuma[3,4] which compared rates of gastrointestinal infection in infants who were exclusively breastfed (for either three or six months or longer), reported that such infections occurred in 7.4% of infants receiving three months' exclusive breastfeeding compared to 5.0% of infants who were exclusively breastfed for six months. They also reported that there were no significant differences between study groups for hospital admissions due to gastrointestinal infections, suggesting that (in their cohort) the duration and exclusivity of breastfeeding did not reduce the risk of more serious gastrointestinal infections. When the time periods of birth to three months, three to six months, and longer than six months' exclusive breastfeeding were considered, the beneficial effect on infections was only evident in the three-to-six-month period. Subsequent follow-up of the cohort has not reported any long-term gastrointestinal ill health.

In the Dundee Infant Feeding Study which was undertaken in the late 1980s and published in the *British Medical Journal* in 1990, 1993 and 1998,[5-7] the analysis on the relationship of breastfeeding to gastrointestinal illness noted that significant confounding variables for this outcome were father's socio-economic status, maternal age, and whether either or both parents smoked. After adjustment for these factors there was no significant difference in gastrointestinal illness between those infants who were exclusively breastfed or were predominantly breastfed for thirteen weeks or longer. When these groups were combined the mean rate of gastrointestinal infection was 4% of infants and in comparison, the never-breastfed group and the breastfed-for-less-than-thirteen-weeks group was 15.7% and 16.7%, respectively. For the infants who were observed throughout the first year of life, thirty-five (5.7%) were admitted to hospital with gastrointestinal illness and the group who were exclusively or predominantly breast fed for thirteen weeks or more had a hospital admission rate for gastrointestinal illness of 2% and for those infants not breastfed or for less than thirteen weeks the rate was 7.8%. It was concluded from this data that receiving breastmilk either exclusively or predominantly for more than thirteen weeks reduces the incidence of gastrointestinal illness during the first year of life. However, as previously noted, the Kramer and Kakuma systematic review of 2002 was considered by an Expert Consultation.[8] Because the level of protective effect against gastrointestinal infection observed in developed countries, coupled with the known high incidence of mortality from gastrointestinal infections in many developing country settings, a global recommendation for exclusive breastfeeding for six months was agreed.

The Expert Consultation concluded that they support a policy of exclusive breastfeeding for six months, with the introduction of complementary foods and continued breastfeeding thereafter, but they also highlighted that these recommendations apply to *populations* – as distinct from individual infants and their families. They further emphasized that some infants will be at risk of nutrient deficiency with six months of exclusive breastfeeding. They also advised that priority must be given to investigating these outcomes in infants who are born 'small for gestational age'. In relation to mothers, it was recommended that further data on breastmilk production and composition from mothers with a body mass index (BMI) of less than 18.5 should be obtained, and that the adequacy of breastmilk for meeting infant requirements to the age of six months should be assessed.

They indicated that the proportion of infants who are exclusively breastfed for six months can be maximized if any potential problems are addressed, including:

- the nutritional status of pregnant and lactating mothers
- the micronutrient status of infants living in areas with a high prevalence of deficiencies (such as iron, zinc and vitamin A)
- the need for routine primary healthcare of individual infants, including assessment of their growth and clinical signs of micronutrient deficiencies.

It is therefore important to note that the original decision by the Expert Consultation to recommend six months exclusive breastfeeding was subject to several important clinical and research caveats, which were not highlighted when the WHO published their *Global Strategy for Infant and Young Child Feeding* in 2003.[9]

Interface between exclusive breastfeeding and the introduction of complementary foods

The interface between exclusive breastfeeding and the introduction of complementary foods has become the flashpoint of infant-feeding policymaking, with WHO and breastfeeding activist groups strongly defending six months' exclusive breastfeeding aligning with introduction of complementary foods at six months. The dilemma is that the evidence for such a precise switch in feeding practice is more subjective than objective and does not allow for normal infant developmental variation.

Gastrointestinal illnesses in developed countries occur less frequently and are milder and more short-lived than those in less developed countries. The difference in incidence of mild gastrointestinal illness between infants receiving six months and three to six months of exclusive breastfeeding is less than 3% for all infants. With this marginal difference in the risk of gastrointestinal illness in developed countries, it is important to equate the risk of not receiving six months of breastmilk exclusively with the potential risks of delaying the introduction of complementary foods to six months.

The Expert Consultation highlighted the importance of the transition period between exclusive breastfeeding and complementary feeding and the risk of nutritional deficiency. They supported complementary feeding at six months, but also recommended the development and evaluation of interventions for micronutrient intake through supplements or complementary foods in different areas of the world. This evaluation would include formative studies to identify processing methods, preparation methods, and the local ingredients required to prepare nutritionally adequate, safe and appropriate complementary foods.

Unfortunately, uncertainty about the optimum timing for introducing complementary foods continues. A position paper by the European Society for Paediatric Gastroenterology, Hepatology and Nutrition (ESPGHAN), published in 2017, stated that exclusive breastfeeding should be promoted for at least four to six months, and that complementary foods (solids and liquids other than breastmilk or infant formula) should not be introduced before four months – and not delayed beyond six months.[10]

Following a request from the European Commission, the European Food Safety Authority requested that the Panel on Nutrition, Novel Foods and Food Allergens (NDA) revised its scientific opinion of 2009 on the appropriate age range for the introduction of complementary feeding into an infant's diet. The review was published in 2019 and concluded that the earliest developmental skills of infants relevant for consuming pureéd complementary foods can be observed between three and four months of age.[11] Some infants have the skills for consuming finger foods at four months, but more commonly at five to seven months. The fact that an infant may be ready from a neurodevelopmental perspective to progress to a more diversified diet before six months of age does not imply that there is a need to introduce complementary foods. Saying that, it is important to be aware of the risks of failing to start complementary foods at six months, because the delay can lead to nutritional deficiency and faltering growth, which may then progress to physical and cognitive stunting.

One option to resolve the stakeholder controversy of duration of exclusive breastfeeding versus the timing of introduction of solid foods, is to be guided by the infant. We do not insist that all infants worldwide start walking at the same age, we allow individual developmental variation to decide, and maybe this should be applied to the variation in infant feeding patterns, with acknowledgement by adults that on this issue, the infant may know best (see Chapter 5).

Breastfeeding for two years or beyond

The phrase 'breastfeeding for two years or beyond' can be traced back to the Innocenti Declaration at the *Policymakers Meeting: Breastfeeding in the 1990s A Global Initiative*, held at the Innocenti Centre in Florence on 30 July 1990.[12] The meeting included representation from thirty countries, of which only three were high-income. Organizational representation included UNICEF, WHO, USAID, the FAO and the World Bank. Although the discussion appears to have been more conversational than scientific, the overriding concern was about children who live in the most difficult circumstances. Despite the differing risks between developing and developed countries, the Declaration recommended breastfeeding for two years or beyond for every child worldwide. The lack of evidence for a universal recommendation in 1990 – and subsequently – has not deterred this statement being a fixture in all infant-feeding policies since that point. The evidence base for universality remains weak, so it is not surprising that there is a high level of non-compliance in families who live in developed countries.

As with other aspects of infant feeding, there should be a pragmatic approach to continued breastfeeding. When the Innocenti Declaration agreed that breastfeeding should continue for two years or beyond, the driver for the long period was the high infant mortality rate in low-income countries.[9] There were no specific research data supporting the same duration of continued breastfeeding for all infants worldwide – and this remains the situation today.

Until there are studies that compare continued breastfeeding for one, two and three years – in both high- and low-income settings – the optimal duration will remain speculative, and thus still be a continuing source of debate and division.

The risks and the benefits need to be considered for individual children and their families. By reaching a decision through this process, parents will feel more involved and gain a sense of ownership and be more inclined to engage and comply with the decision.

Based on the current literature, a reasonable suggestion may be two years or beyond for low-income countries, but for some high-income countries and individual families a stepping-stone of one year or beyond may be more realistic. What is most damaging – and should be avoided – is the setting of targets that are excessively aspirational, lack scientific evidence, and lead to disengagement of the target population.

Despite the clear evidence of non-compliance with breastfeeding for two years or beyond, the WHO seemed to be in a state of denial when it made the recommendation, in 2016, that milk products marketed for children up to the age of three years should be understood to be breastmilk substitutes.[13] Why was this statement made when the evidence was clear that the vast majority of mothers were not breastfeeding during the third year of life, and these products were therefore not substituting breastmilk? The intervention appears to lack insight and good sense.

Moreover, the WHO need to appreciate that increasing the recommended duration of breastfeeding to three years increases the legitimacy of marketing and sales opportunities for infant formula companies. Not surprisingly, there is now an increasing number of formulas specifically 'designed' for infants during the first, second and third years of life, thus further fuelling the buoyant formula market. Rather than putting so much focus on a liquid diet in early life, they should be ensuring that all infants receive nutritious complementary foods during this period, and ultimately will have progressed to a nutritious family diet by the age of three years.

Finally, an important non-nutritional consideration is that breastfeeding causes maternal amenorrhoea and infertility during the period of breastfeeding, and it is therefore important to note that prolonged breastfeeding may therefore be associated with a longer period of infertility.[14] Parents need to consider what they believe is appropriate for them as a family; how do they view the potential benefits or risks of prolonged breastfeeding against the potential benefits or risks of prolonged periods of reduced fertility? To answer these questions parents need to be provided with the best evidence. The drive to encourage mothers to breastfeed during the third year of their child's life needs to be balanced against the implications of the robust scientific evidence demonstrating a direct causation between breastfeeding and infertility, and this needs to be balanced against the data on 'associations' between breastfeeding and several other health conditions, including breast cancer. It is important that organizations such as WHO present advice to parents that clearly separates hypothetical potential mechanisms of possible causation from tried and tested mechanisms that clearly demonstrate evidence of causation (see Chapter 11).

Personalized breastmilk and depersonalized infant-feeding policies

Many articles on breastfeeding begin by stating that breastmilk has evolved over many thousands of years, and thus should be considered the ideal source of nutrition for all newborn infants. Biological evolution refers to the cumulative changes that occur in a population over time, with the changes taking place at a genetic level, as genes mutate and/or recombine in different ways during reproduction and are passed on to future generations. Through this process, individuals may inherit new characteristics that give them a survival or reproductive advantage in their local environments. This is referred to as natural selection.[15,16] For example, individuals who are able to access nutritional foods live longer, on average, and produce more offspring than those who are less able. Applying this theory to breastfeeding, it is postulated that the content of breastmilk is the culmination of many genetically driven changes in response to adverse environmental factors. Therefore the composition of breastmilk is assumed to enhance the survival needs of individual infants and young children.

Although there may be some justification for stating that the Darwinian theory of evolution is responsible for breastmilk being the ideal food source for all infants, it has been suggested that a broader interpretation of the theory is that the mother–child dyad is the 'evolutionary unit'. And to ensure the survival of *Homo sapiens*, both mother and child (and probably the whole family unit) need to benefit from evolutionary changes.[15,16]

This perspective highlights the importance of viewing infant-feeding policy within the context of the needs of a family, whereby breastfeeding is one of several adaptive factors that generate genetic and non-genetic influences on survival and wellbeing within populations. This concept of multifactorial evolutionary change may be helpful for understanding why a 'one size fits all' global infant-feeding policy may lack sensitivity and specificity for sections of the global population.

There is a marked variation in the composition of breastmilk, which has been extensively documented.[17] The compositional differences can be identified at different points during the lactation period. For example, there are wide variations in the content of key vitamins such as B_6, B_{12} and vitamin C, which tend to decline with the duration of breastfeeding. Calcium, iron, zinc and copper concentrations also gradually decrease throughout the period of lactation. Fat composition displays large inter- and intra-individual variation among lactating mothers, depending on the duration of lactation and the time of day, as well as during each breastfeeding session.

The relationship of maternal diet to infant nutrition, both before and after birth, undoubtedly contributes to the marked inter- and intra-variability of breastmilk composition across populations.[17] Vitamin B12 levels, for example, have been shown to correlate with the mothers' diet, with lower concentrations in the milk of vegetarian mothers compared to omnivorous mothers. Vitamin K and vitamin D concentrations in human milk are generally considered to be insufficient, and it is recommended that infants should be supplemented at birth. The long-chain polyunsaturated fatty acid (PUFA) content of the maternal diet, especially docosahexaenoic acid (DHA), relates to the levels within breastmilk, and these may influence infant cognitive, visual and immunological function.

This catalogue of nutrient variability during lactation can be presented as the consequence of natural selection determining optimum nutrition for individual infants, or it could be interpreted as evidence of breastmilk composition being susceptible to many external nutritive and non-nutritive factors, with positive or negative influences. Policy-makers and breastfeeding advocates are sympathetic to the former advocating the concept of 'personalized medicine',[18] but it is clear that there is no one-size-fits-all construct for milk composition that can inform optimal 'personalized' human milk for specific settings and contexts.

Moreover, policy-makers need to explain how these continuous changes in the composition of breastmilk align with the rigid, one-size-fits-all approach to WHO's policy on the timing of breastmilk consumption. This would appear to be another paradox, where the consumption of 'personalized' breastmilk is controlled by a depersonalized infant-feeding policy. Would it not make more sense to personalize the whole infant-feeding process, with personalized breastmilk consumed according to the personal need of each infant? Who knows best – the infant or the policy-maker?

It is evident that the marketing and promotion of breastfeeding is complex and, as a consequence, key messages may appear questionable and paradoxical in nature. Examples of common paradoxical statements and their related explanations are shown in Table 4.1 (*overpage*).

Table 4.1: Eight paradoxes of infant feeding.

Paradox	Explanation
1. Breastfeeding duration is longer in countries with the highest rates of maternal mortality, infant and child mortality, malnutrition and stunting.	The adverse effect of other nutritional and non-nutritional factors on infant and child morbidity and mortality exceeds the potential health benefits of breastmilk.
2. Emerging economies with rising consumption of infant formula have rapidly reducing infant mortality.	In these countries the health benefits of other nutritional and non-nutritional developments exceed the potential adverse effects of infant formulas.
3. The many years of evolutionary change are associated with considerable inter- and intra-variability of breastmilk composition.	Evolutionary change takes place within populations, and the genetic drivers for increased survival and wellbeing differ between populations.
4. Variations in maternal diet can lead to marked variation in breastmilk composition.	Evolutionary changes in maternal diet can have a direct effect on breastmilk composition, which may provide beneficial or harmful effects on the infant.
5. The introduction of solid foods is considered to be complementary to breastmilk.	The quality of infant and young-child diets depends on the quality of both breastmilk and available solid foods; these sources of nutrition should be mutually complementary.
6. Breastmilk is considered to be a personalized medicine.	The composition of breastmilk is personalized by maternal diet, cultural, ethnic, genetic and geographical factors and is therefore family-specific (and may or may not be beneficial).
7. Breastmilk is personalized, but infant-feeding policy is depersonalized.	The variations in breastmilk composition are presented as personalized and beneficial, but policy-makers have decided that the timings for the consumption of breastmilk and complementary foods are depersonalized and inflexible.
8. Surveys on maternal reasons for ceasing breastfeeding rarely mention industry marketing of infant formulas.	The predominant reasons provided by parents are that they believe they are not providing sufficient milk for their infant and when experiencing difficulties advice and support are inadequate.

Clearly there is a need for scientific evidence to explain the paradox of personalized breastfeeding, in terms of breastmilk composition, but depersonalized by universal policy recommendations. Policy-makers have (controversially) adopted infant-feeding policies that do not allow variation, and they have attempted to introduce legislation and sanctions to cement their rigid thinking on this matter.

Note that the fat concentration in breastmilk more than doubles between the time of birth and two years of lactation. The reason that has been offered for this shift is that the additional fat intake increases energy intake during a period of rapid growth.[17] But this does not explain the paradoxical reduction in carbohydrate intake, the alternative energy source. And during this time, of course, the child will be receiving significant energy and nutrient intake in the form of solid foods. This highlights the importance of not considering the composition of breastmilk in isolation. Reference must be made to the composition of complementary foods – which then raises the issue of the optimum timing for introducing solid foods.

Disentangling the relationships between breastmilk composition and consumption, complementary food composition and consumption, and policy decisions on the introduction and duration of both of these sources of food, is required if validity of the current policy is going to be achieved. In the meantime, a one-size-fits-all policy will continue to be considered with suspicion, and compliance will remain a problem.

Breastmilk and the newborn gastrointestinal tract

During pregnancy the main nutritional supply to the fetus is from the mother through the umbilical cord, although during the prenatal period infants swallow amniotic fluid which aids the development of the gut and provides approximately 10–15% of their nutritional intake. At birth the gastrointestinal tract is still very immature from an anatomical, physiological and immunological perspective, and for this reason the way an infant is fed from birth can have significant health implications.

Breastmilk has many properties that allow the gastrointestinal tract to develop during this period. Nutritionally, breastfeeding provides biologically human nutrients produced by the mother, which are accompanied by factors that aid digestion, including specific enzymes such as human milk lipase. From an immunological perspective there are many factors that may provide protection to infants.

Among these are immunoglobulins (secretory IgA) against microbes to which the mother has been exposed, antibacterial and antiviral agents (like lactoferrin, lysozyme and certain fatty acids); and oligosaccharides, which act by blocking pathogens or bacteria from binding to human cells. All of these components allow the normal gut flora (*Bifidobacteria* and *Lactobacilli*) to colonize the gut and enhance the gastrointestinal and immunological functions of the infant.

This evidence strongly supports the policy that all infants should be attached to the breast shortly after birth to initiate the supply of the immunological components (in colostrum) and stimulate the lactation process. With the right support, and appropriate realistic messages for parents on breastfeeding, this should be achievable for the vast majority of parents. From a health-professional perspective, there should be an incremental process of encouragement and support, but at all times the views of parents should be respected. As discussed, there is evidence that the recommended durations of exclusive and continuing breastfeeding are not within the range of most parents, and it is difficult to persuade parents of this guidance when much of the evidence remains equivocal. There is, however, good enough evidence to encourage mothers to exclusively breastfeed for at least four to six months, then partially breastfeed thereafter. In almost all publications that provide a reference for six months' exclusive breastfeeding, the authors highlight that their study was limited because it was difficult to determine whether the infants were actually exclusively breastfed or predominantly or partially breastfed. Interestingly, this applies to the high-profile study by Victora and colleagues, who reported that scaling-up breastfeeding to a near-universal level could prevent 823,000 deaths a year in children younger than five years.[18] The calculation for lives saved included an analysis of partial breastfeed versus no breastfeeding the former being because of the lack of clarity on infants who were exclusively or predominantly breastfed.

A 'rule of thumb' should be that the initial months of breastfeeding will provide greater health benefit to the child than the last months of breastfeeding (whenever they are), and therefore the focus should be on the former.

Suboptimal lactation

Many studies have reported on the reasons that mothers cease breastfeeding. Maternal responses tend to identify basic preventable healthcare issues, such as the management of breast pain, concerns about adequacy of milk supply, and a perception that their infant is not satiated. In addition, there are lifestyle, health and socioeconomic factors that may have an impact on the initiation and continuance of breastfeeding. However, many mothers believe the fundamental issue is that they do not produce a sufficient quantity of breastmilk.

In practice, it has been assumed that breastfeeding is a natural biological process that enables all mothers to provide sufficient milk for their infant,[18] but this is being increasingly challenged, with a recent claim that chronic lactation insufficiency is a significant public health issue.

Shere and colleagues define chronic lactation insufficiency as the production of less milk than is required to exclusively feed an infant for the duration of the breastfeeding period, despite following best practices.[19] Several of the authors of this paper are founding members of the newly launched Low Milk Supply Foundation, a non-profit organization dedicated to addressing the gap in research and knowledge relating to chronic lactation insufficiency. It is estimated that 5–15% of breastfeeding mothers experience this insufficiency. In the USA alone, this would equate to 180,000 to 500,000 breastfeeding dyads per year.

The lactating breast would be unique among glandular organs if there were not some variations in function between breastfeeding mothers. Issues with organ function occur throughout the body, and within the reproductive system, where there is the potential for failure of conception, placental dysfunction and abnormal parturition. Therefore lactation failure in some mothers should not be unexpected.

It has long been assumed that once lactation is successfully initiated, the primary factor regulating milk production is infant demand. This is why interventions have focused on improving breastfeeding education and early lactation support. However, in addition to other factors (including maternal nutrition and hormonal regulation), there is an increasing array of maternal genetic and modifiable factors, such as diet and environmental exposures, which may influence reproductive endocrinology and lactation physiology.[20]

A recent review by Boss and colleagues considered evidence on the availability of methods for objectively assessing lactation. The authors introduced the topic, noting that:

> "… basic research into the physiology and biochemistry of the lactating human mammary gland is limited, and there have been no major advances toward the assessment of its normal function in recent times".[20]

They further commented that the breast is unlike other major organs, such as the heart, brain, liver, lungs and kidneys, for which there is an array of objective tests for assessing function. But with lactation, the authors point out, there are no well-defined parameters for measuring normal human lactation (other than measuring infant growth).

The assessment of the success of lactation is usually based on general health evidence, on factors such as a lack of discomfort, a perception by mothers that their milk supply is adequate and having no concerns relating to infant and maternal health. In such circumstances, 'medicalizing' breastfeeding would be unwise. But what should the clinical input be if there *are* concerns about a mother's milk supply? Or about infant weight gain and increasing maternal anxiety about infant satiety?

The current response would be to reassure mothers that all women can successfully breastfeed their infant. The healthcare input would focus on the breastfeeding process, rather than considering that there may be an inherent biological difficulty with lactation.[21] With 5–15% of mothers believing they are unable to provide sufficient milk for their infants, and with potential physical consequences for the infants and well-documented emotional and psychological consequences for mothers, should sub-optimal lactation be considered as a clinical condition and therefore be treated in a similar fashion to sub-optimal cardiac, respiratory or renal function? This is discussed further in Chapter 11.

Emotional and psychological consequences of ceasing breastfeeding

It is most unusual for a mother to change to infant formula if she is successfully breastfeeding. Moreover, maternal surveys indicate that the marketing and promotion of infant formula is a surprisingly unusual reason for cessation.

In one of the most extensive surveys, thirty-two factors were identified that contribute to the cessation of breastfeeding. None related to issues regarding the advertising or promotion of infant formulas. The most significant factors were lactational, nutritional, psychosocial and lifestyle. The authors concluded that it is necessary to address these challenges and support mothers to achieve their desired breastfeeding outcome.[22] It is argued that infant-formula companies have a large budget for promoting their products, but it must also be acknowledged that health expenditure on advising and supporting *every* woman who is having a baby on *all* aspects of breastfeeding during the antenatal and postnatal periods is considerable and will undoubtedly exceed any industry promotion and marketing expenditure on infant formulas. From a health-authority perspective, there is a requirement to ensure that the health budget is available, and that it is effectively and efficiently utilized to provide the best infant feeding care for mothers and infants.

A common concern expressed by parents is the lack of support at critical times – a significant contributor to premature breastfeeding cessation. A key element of parental support is providing them with a realistic view regarding both the enjoyment of and potential woes of breastfeeding. They need to be adequately prepared for these experiences. Psychosociologists have been highlighting the importance of self-efficacy during breastfeeding, that is the individual's belief in his or her capacity to execute behaviours and have the ability to reach specific performance attainments.[23] This involves developing confidence in their ability to control their own motivation, behaviour and social environment.

A systematic review of the psychosocial correlates of exclusive breastfeeding focused on factors that may enable mothers to achieve exclusive breastfeeding for six months. The authors concluded that psychological factors are highly predictive of exclusive-breastfeeding outcomes, and that these factors may be sensitive to interventions and experiences and thus influence the duration of breastfeeding.[23]

However, there are limitations currently on the available data, mainly because researchers have adopted different methodologies in their studies. For example, the definitions of exclusive breastfeeding are varied, and sample sizes are small. Two personal anecdotal accounts are shown in Box 4.1 (*overpage*), that reflect the contrasting experiences of some mothers. Whatever their circumstances and views, it is important for parents to feel that the practice of feeding their infant is within their control from the first feed.[24] Any advice maybe perceived as 'pressure', and with pressure comes anxiety and loss of confidence. A mother's emotional turmoil can extend to their partner and other family members, who offer their own advice too.

The first letter in Box 4.1 is an example of a mother who comes to a point of realization that the only way she can take back control over feeding her child is to cease breastfeeding and commence formula. This situation must be avoided.

Box 4.1: Mothers' attitudes to infant feeding—published letters

The Guardian Weekend (4 January 2020)
A LETTER TO THE LACTATION CONSULTANT

"As a stay-at-home mum, you have the time you need to figure this out." That was what you said after I explained that I was spending twelve hours a day feeding my son – trying to breastfeed him, giving him a bottle when he was still hungry after the feeding, pumping up after that, washing the pump parts, mixing up the formula, and then starting the whole process over again. I was overwhelmed.

"How long have you been using the hospital-grade pump?"

"Have you tried the nipple shield?"

"Have you fixed his tongue tie?"

"How much fenugreek are you taking?"

"Have you been eating lots of garlic?"

I did all those things and more, and you were still convinced that the solution was more time and effort from me. *"Women were designed to breastfeed! Shouldn't a stay-at-home mum be willing to spend all her waking hours doing it?"*

I just needed to buck up and realise that being a mother requires sacrifice and hard work. You didn't say these things in those exact words, but you implied them.

One day I realised I was spending more time thinking about how to breastfeed my son than anything else. It was consuming everything. And your urgings reminded me there was always more I could do … more fenugreek, more lactation cookies, more mother's milk tea, more essential oils, more water, more calories, more nutritious calories, more hand expression … more, more, more.

But I was also feeling more anxious. I didn't feel a deep, close bond with my baby. I second-guessed everything I was doing. I felt incompetent. I didn't have much time to enjoy him. My milk supply didn't increase.

So I quit breastfeeding. Today I am a happy stay-at-home mum who spends my days feeding my baby, playing with him, doing his laundry, reading to him, and enjoying him. The long days at home as my baby's primary caregiver did give me the time to figure things out and for me that meant switching to a bottle. I don't regret it.

The path you were pushing me on was one where I focused on my own efforts and judged myself on how they turned out. But in motherhood, as in life, you can't always control the outcome, so my focus is now on doing the best I can. I wasn't able to 'figure out' breastfeeding, but I was able to figure out something about being a mother.

The Guardian (26 April 2019)
A MOTHER'S RESPONSE TO AN ARTICLE ON BREASTFEEDING

I think perhaps this debate has got a bit out of hand. I had four babies, my older sister had five, and our younger sister had three. For a variety of reasons, some of these babies were breastfed, some were bottle-fed, and some a combination of the two. But I don't recall any of us having nervous breakdowns about decisions made. Making personal choices on rational grounds is part of being an adult, and definitely part of being a parent.

Perhaps sensible mums will check out the pros and cons, ignore the pressure groups and doom merchant, face the realities of the situation, stop being bullied by ideas of 'perfection' and just get on with it.

Approaches to breastfeeding have to be sensitive, relaxed and realistic as indicated in the second letter. Interventions that enhance self-efficacy may engender sufficient confidence and motivation to maintain control and enjoyment of the breastfeeding experience, which the mother can then share with others.

Personalized care and support for parents

In developing an infant feeding strategy for an individual infant and family, it is important to ensure there is a common understanding of the key objectives of the feeding plan, with consideration of the potential positive and negative outcomes. Appropriate solutions should be identified and agreed. This approach should ensure that there are no surprises for the parents, that they are prepared for difficulties that may arise, and that they are aware of the potential changes that may be required to the feeding plan.

It is preferable for these decisions to be made with local health professionals whom they know and trust, especially because knowledge of the family circumstances will inform the health professionals' judgement and management of any feeding issues.[25]

A key element of this approach is that there must be acceptance that solutions may include partial breastfeeding, or stopping breastfeeding, or introducing infant formula and starting complementary foods. The need to change from WHO's recommended practice should not be considered by parents or health professionals as a 'failure' – and should not be delayed to a point at which an infant is unwell and the mother's emotional and psychological issues are dominant.

The balance between infant feeding and maternal health concerns must be carefully considered, and it may be that individual clinical judgements may override global policy. This approach runs contrary to the current WHO prospectus of no deviation from a rigid one-dimensional policy, but a more flexible approach may resonate with the conclusions from a recent systematic review of the Baby Friendly Initiative (BFI) in the UK.[26] The authors' key findings acknowledged that support is highly influential to women's experiences of BFI-compliant care, but the current provision:

> "… may promote unrealistic expectations of breastfeeding, not meet women's individual needs, and may foster negative emotional experiences".

A systematic review of twenty published papers, conducted by the same research group, explored guilt and/or shame in relation to infant-feeding outcomes. It concluded that guilt is experienced more frequently when breastfeeding exclusivity and other breastfeeding intentions are unmet.[27] For breastfeeding mothers, the guilt relates to family and peers, while for formula-feeding mothers the guilt relates to healthcare professionals and peers. The authors of the review noted that there is limited data on the relation of shame with infant-feeding outcomes, so further research is required. The authors also recommended supplying more realistic, non-judgemental and mother-centred support to minimize guilt and shame. They also suggested that a shift in messaging from 'six months exclusive breastfeeding' to 'every feed counts' may be more receptive.

In conclusion, there is evidence that emotional and psychological symptoms relating to the reduction or cessation of breastfeeding need to be mitigated. This may be achieved by carefully agreeing individual infant feeding plans that align with scientific evidence and reflect the needs of infants as well as the wishes of parents. There should also be options for addressing potential breastfeeding difficulties, in order to prevent feelings of failure. Most importantly, the overall objective should be to enable all parents to be able to reflect on the feeding of their infant as an enjoyable and fulfilling experience whether their infants are breastfed, partially breastfed or formula fed.

A key message for policy-makers should be that policies need to be viewed by parents as *achievable*. The psychosocial consequences of overreaching targets are not only a *dis*incentive but may also be physically and emotionally harmful. The extremes of idealistic 'wishful' thinking and the harsh reality of coping with a newborn infant in difficult socioeconomic circumstances need to be factored into a workable solution for both parents and their children. This is particularly important for mothers from families that have no previous experience of breastfeeding, and whose infants would benefit most from the health effects of breastmilk. In difficult circumstances like these, the policy message should be:

- to 'give it a try'
- to initially consider breastfeeding duration in weeks rather than months or years
- to recognize that every additional week of breastfeeding has the potential to provide additional health benefit to the child, and – ultimately –
- to assess the achievement of the breastfeeding experience within the context of the parents' families and community.

A balanced incremental approach may allow the development of a greater sense of ownership and confidence which may mitigate the sense of overwhelming pressure and failure, and consequently redefine the essence of a successful breastfeeding experience.

Conclusion

In 2018 the WHO expressed concern (in Resolution 71.9) about the following:[28]

- nearly two in every three infants aged under six months of age are not exclusively breastfed
- in high-income countries, fewer than one in five infants are breastfed for twelve months
- in low- and middle-income countries, only two in every three children between six months and two years of age receive any breastmilk.

The WHO position – that infant and young-child feeding policies should be universal – is undoubtedly challenging for parents, as well as for health professionals. Families living in high-income countries fully appreciate the risks faced by families living with no clean water, poor sanitation, shortages of nutritious foods, and limited health and educational support. For vulnerable families, prolonged breastfeeding is essential. But it has to be recognized that the poorest countries have not only the longest duration of breastfeeding but also the highest rates of childhood mortality and stunting of growth. This is associated with an insufficiency of nutritious complementary foods, and in these circumstances, breastmilk is an inadequate complementary food substitute. Infant and young-child nutrition should be personalized to meet the nutritional requirements of each child, and this will differ for high-, medium- and low-income families. The priority for parents in each of these categories is that the feeding regimen should meet their child's needs and be provided safely within their community.

Addendum

This chapter is based on a previously published article: Forsyth JS (2011) Policy and pragmatism in breastfeeding. *Archives of Diseases in Childhood* 96, 909–10.

References

1. Fewtrell M, Wilson DC, Booth I, *et al.* (2010) Six months of exclusive breastfeeding: how good is the evidence? *British Medical Journal* 342, c5955. DOI: 10.1136/bmj. c5955.

2. WHO (2011) WHO Media Centre Statement, 15 January 2011. *Exclusive breast-feeding for six months best for babies everywhere.* Available at: https://www.who. int/news/item/15-01-2011-exclusive-breastfeeding-for-six-months-best-for-babies-everywhere (last accessed July 2022).

3. Kramer MS, Kakuma R (2002) Optimal duration of exclusive breastfeeding. *Cochrane Database of Systematic Reviews* 20128, CD003517. DOI: 10.1002/14651858.CD003517. PMID: 11869667. Available at: https://pubmed.ncbi.nlm.nih.gov/11869667/ (last accessed August 2022).

4. Kramer MS, Kakuma R (2012) Optimal duration of exclusive breastfeeding. *Cochrane Database of Systematic Reviews* CD003517. DOI: 10.1002/14651858.CD003517.pub2.PMID: 22895934.

5. Howie PW, Forsyth S, Ogston SA, *et al.* (1990) Protective effect of breast feeding against infection. *British Medical Journal* 300, 11–16.

6. Forsyth S, Ogston SA, Clark A, *et al.* (1993) Relation between early introduction of solid food to infants and their weight and illnesses during the first two years of life. *British Medical Journal* 306, 1572–76.

7. Wilson AC, Forsyth JS, Greene SA, *et al.* (1998) Relation of infant diet to childhood health: seven-year follow-up of a cohort of children in the Dundee infant feeding study. *British Medical Journal* 316, 21–25.

8. WHO (2001) *Report of the Expert Consultation on the optimal duration of exclusive breastfeeding.* Available at: https://apps.who.int/iris/bitstream/handle/10665/67219/WHO_NHD_01.09.pdf?ua=1 (last accessed August (2022).

9. WHO (2003) *Global strategy for infant and young-child feeding.* Available at: http://whqlibdoc.who.int/publications/2003/9241562218.pdf (last accessed August 2022).

10. Fewtrell M, Bronsky I, Campoy C, *et al.* (2017) Complementary feeding: A position paper by the ESPGHAN Committee on Nutrition. *Journal of Paediatric Gastroenterology and Nutrition* 64, 119–32.

11. Castenmiller J, de Henauw S, Hirsch-Ernst K, *et al.* (European Food Safety Authority NDA Panel) (2019) Scientific Opinion on the appropriate age range for introduction of complementary feeding into an infant's diet. *EFSA Journal* 17, 5780.

12. UNICEF (2006) *Celebrating the Innocenti Declaration on the protection, promotion and support of breastfeeding 1990–2005.* UNICEF Innocenti Research Centre.

13. Grummer-Strawn LM (2018) Clarifying the definition of breastmilk substitutes. *Journal of Pediatric Gastroenterology and Nutrition* 67, 683

14. McNeilly A (1969) Breastfeeding and the suppression of fertility. *Food and Nutrition Bulletin* 17, 163,

15. Dugdale AE (1986) Evolution and infant feeding. *The Lancet* 1, 670–73.

16. Cuthbertson WFJ (1999) Evolution of infant nutrition. *British Journal of Nutrition* 81, 359–71.

17. Dror K, Allen LH (2018) Overview of nutrients in human milk. *Advances in Nutrition* 9, 278S–94S.

18. Victora CG, Bahl R, Barros AJD, *et al.* (2016) Breastfeeding in the 21st century: epidemiology, mechanisms, and lifelong effect. *The Lancet* 38, 475–90.

19. Shere H, Weijer L, Dashnow H, *et al.* (2021) Chronic lactation insufficiency is a public health issue: Commentary on 'We need patient-centered research in breastfeeding medicine' by Stuebe. *Breastfeeding Medicine* 16, 349–50. DOI: 10.1089/bfm.2021.0202.

20. Boss M, Gardner H, Hartmann P (2018) Normal human lactation: closing the gap. *F1000 Research 7F1000 Faculty Reviews* 8019.

21. Lee S, Kelleher SL (2016) Biological underpinnings of breastfeeding challenges: the role of genetics, diet, and environment on lactation physiology. *American Journal of Physiology Endocrinology and Metabolism* 311, E405–22. DOI:10.1152/ajpendo.00495.2015.

22. Odom EC, Li R, Scanlon KS, Perrine CG, Grummer-Strawn L (2013) Reasons for earlier than desired cessation of breastfeeding. *Pediatrics* 131, e726–32.

23. Galipeau R, Baillot A, Trottier A, Lemire L (2018) Effectiveness of interventions on breastfeeding self-efficacy and perceived insufficient milk supply: A systematic review and meta-analysis. *Maternal and Child Nutrition* 14, e12607,

24. Jackson L, De Pascalis L, Harrold J, Fallon V (2021) Guilt, shame, and postpartum infant feeding outcomes: A systematic review. *Maternal and Child Nutrition* 17, e13141.

25. Hoddinott P, Craig LCA, Britten J, *et al.* (2012) A serial qualitative interview study of infant feeding experiences. *BMJ Open 2*, e000504. Available at: DOI:10.1136/ https://bmjopen.bmj.com/content/bmjopen/2/2/e000504.full.pdf/ (last accessed August 2022).

26. Fallon VM, Harrold JA, Chisholm A (2019) The impact of the UK Baby Friendly Initiative on maternal and infant health outcomes: A mixed-methods systematic review. *Maternal and Child Nutrition* 153, e12778.

27. Jackson L, De Pascalis L, Harrold J, Fallon V (2021) Guilt, shame, and postpartum infant feeding outcomes: A systematic review. *Maternal and Child Nutrition* 17, e13141.

28. WHA (2018) *Infant and young child feeding. WHA 71.9. Agenda item 12.6 26 (May 2018).* Available at: (https://www.who.int/news/item/15-01-2011-exclusive-breastfeeding-for-six-months-best-for-babies-everywhere (last accessed February 2022).

CHAPTER 5

Why has complementary feeding been neglected?

In early life, infant and young children require a continuous supply of optimal nutrition to meet their energy and nutrient requirements during a critically important period of growth and development. The key food sources at this time are breastmilk, infant formula (if required), and complementary foods.

Complementary feeding begins when breastmilk alone is no longer sufficient to meet an infant's nutritional requirements, usually around six months of age. To meet energy and nutrient requirements during the complementary feeding period from six months to twenty-four months, it is important that measures are taken to ensure that the nutritional interface between breastfeeding and complementary foods delivers a balanced diet.

The relationship between breastmilk and complementary foods was elegantly presented over twenty years ago in a document published by the WHO.[1] It was estimated that for the period of twelve months to twenty-three months, in infants that receive an average volume of breastmilk, the energy consumed from breastmilk reduces from:

- 413 kcals/day at six to eight months, to
- 379 kcals/day at nine to eleven months, and
- 346 kcals/day at twelve to twenty-three months.

These intake data were used to estimate energy requirements from complementary foods. At twelve to twenty-three months, energy from complementary foods was 746 kcals/day (the latter providing 75% of daily energy requirements). Data for thirty-six months are not available, but it can be assumed that the trend will continue, with a significantly higher energy intake from complementary foods (solids and drinks). In relation to specific nutrients, the daily contribution from complementary foods at twelve months to twenty-three months are shown in Table 5.1 (*overpage*).

Table 5.1: The contribution of nutrients in complementary foods in the infant diet at 12–23 months.

Protein	46%
Iron	97%
Zinc	86%
Phosphorus	71%
Magnesium	78%
Sodium	80%
Calcium	56%
Vitamin D	95%

This clearly demonstrates the importance of complementary feeding for ensuring normal growth and development. As previously mentioned, most countries with the longest duration of breastfeeding also have the highest rates of malnutrition and stunting. This is related to the inadequacy of complementary feeding in these countries, and is a poignant reminder that breastmilk does not have the nutritional capability to act as a complementary food substitute.

A more appropriate description of the relationship between breastfeeding and complementary feeding during the second year of life might be that breastfeeding and foods and drinks complement each other, which reflects the continuing importance of breastfeeding, while also recognizing the overriding need for increased diversity in the diet when there is rapid growth and development.

Complementary-feeding strategy

It is stated in WHO's strategy for infant and young-child feeding and two WHO documents on complementary feeding in the breastfed child (2002) and the non-breastfed child (2005),[2-4] that there should be exclusive breastfeeding for six months and continued breastfeeding for two years or beyond; and complementary foods should be introduced at six months, with a focus on nutrient-rich, home-prepared, locally available products, including animal-source food. This is a worthy aspiration, but not necessarily an achievable goal. For example, a key benefit from breastfeeding (compared to formula milk) is the reduced risk of infection, particularly in communities where there is a lack of clean water and absent or limited sanitation facilities. In these circumstances it is not possible to safely prepare locally available complementary foods, so alternatives must be found. There is strong evidence that making major improvements in housing, water supplies and sanitation facilities reduce the risk of infection and mortality. From a nutrition perspective, however, if an infant cannot receive breastmilk, then the safety net has to be infant formula; and if local nutritious complementary foods are not available (or cannot be safely cooked) then a safety net of an external supply chain of prepared nutritional infant and young-child food products that can be safely consumed, is also required.

The WHO has had a longstanding history of non-cooperation with the infant food industry. This approach is strongly supported by breastfeeding advocacy groups and, as a consequence, there appears to be a reluctance to refresh complementary-feeding policy-making and practice. Past transgressions of the Code have fuelled suspicions that industry will exploit the opportunity to promote complementary food products and breach the current Code and policy recommendations. Industry, in turn, has become wary of breastfeeding advocates and activists, viewing them as potentially hostile to their brand name and business interests. As a result, industry has been hesitant about playing a meaningful role in scaling-up complementary products.

UNICEF captured the dilemma facing policy-makers when they stated:[5]

> *"… following the welcoming of the Guidance on Ending the Inappropriate Promotion of Foods for Infants and Young Children by the WHA in mid-2016, governments should enact legislation and adopt policies to prohibit the inappropriate promotion of all commercially produced food or beverage products that are specifically marketed as suitable for feeding children up to 36 months of age, while continuing to adopt and enforce the International Code of Marketing of Breastmilk Substitutes".*

But they continued:

> *"… the private sector and the food industry in particular must contribute to produce affordable, nutritious complementary foods and comply with legislation and policies in place to control inappropriate promotion of commercially produced foods".*

There is, therefore, an acceptance by UNICEF that industry has a role to play, *provided* they abide by the marketing recommendations.[5] As the past has been dominated by issues relating to breastfeeding, it may be that a focus on complementary foods could allow relationships to develop – relationships that may not only lead to improvements in the provision of safe complementary foods (especially in circumstances where local supplies are inadequate) but also facilitate development of a collective approach. Thus, issues regarding non-compliance with the Code could finally be addressed, but for this to emerge as a cohesive plan, there needs to be consultation, compromise, trust, respect and commitment. Unfortunately, the response to the recent European Food Safety Authority (EFSA) opinion paper on the appropriate age range for introducing complementary foods rapidly dispelled any signs of stakeholders – including WHO – from taking a conciliatory view on policy.[6] This 2019 EFSA review concluded that:

> "... the available data do not allow the determination of a single age for the introduction of complementary foods for infants living in Europe. The appropriate age range depends on the individual's characteristics and development, even more so if the infant was born preterm. As long as the foods are given in an age-appropriate texture, are nutritionally appropriate and prepared according to good hygiene practices, there is no convincing evidence that the introduction of complementary foods is associated with either adverse or beneficial health effects (except for infants at risk of iron depletion) at any age investigated in the included studies. For nutritional reasons, the majority of infants need complementary foods from around 6 months of age, and for preterm infants this refers to post-term age. Infants at risk of iron depletion exclusively breastfed infants born to mothers with low iron status, or with early umbilical cord clamping (within 1 minute after birth), or born preterm, or born small for gestational age (SGA) or with high growth velocity, may benefit from introduction of complementary foods that are a source of iron before 6 months of age".

During the public consultation of the draft document there were responses from a range of organizations with strong breastfeeding interests including WHO, Baby Milk Action Europe, IBFAN and First Steps Nutrition Trust. Many concerns were expressed, but the fundamental issue for them was that allowing complementary foods to be offered before six months is not in alignment with the policy of exclusive breastfeeding for six months. What EFSA is reporting is that there is no evidence of harm if solid foods are introduced between four and six months, but they are not specifically recommending that there should be a policy to do so. What policy-makers need to do is consider whether greater flexibility around the six months' time point may resolve this policy conflict.

Insights into the views of WHO were provided in the consultation process of the EFSA paper. Their key statements, published by their colleagues at Baby Milk Action, are considered in Box 5.1.[7]

Box 5.1: Key statements from WHO in the consultation process of the EFSA paper[7]

WHO STATEMENT 1

"A recent systematic review by the US Departments of Agriculture and Health and Human Services came to the conclusion that 'introduction of complementary foods and beverages before age 4 months may be associated with higher odds of overweight/obesity'. There is, therefore, at least some evidence of harm from early introduction of complementary foods."

Author's comments: The results of the systematic review by the US Departments of Agriculture and Health and Human Services are as follows:

*"Eighty-one articles were included in this systematic review that addressed timing of complementary foods and beverages (CFBs) introduction relative to growth, size and body-composition outcomes from infancy through adulthood. Moderate evidence suggests that introduction of CFBs between the ages of 4 and 5 months compared with ~ 6 months is **not** [author's emphasis] associated with differences in weight status, body composition, body circumferences, weight or length among generally healthy, full-term infants. Limited evidence suggests that introduction of CFBs **before** [author's emphasis] age 4 months may be associated with higher odds of overweight/ obesity. Insufficient evidence exists regarding introduction at age ≥ 7 months".*

Author's comments: The US systematic review fits with the general view that complementary feeding at four to five months does not increase the risk of obesity, and introduction before 4 months is not recommended.

WHO STATEMENT 2

"The EFSA Panel concluded that there is no evidence that the introduction of complementary foods before 6 months of age increases gastrointestinal infections. This stands in direct contrast to the conclusion of a previous Cochrane review that concluded 'infants who continue exclusive breastfeeding for 6 months or more appear to have a significantly reduced risk of gastrointestinal infection'."

Author's comments: The evidence on infant gastrointestinal illness relates to the duration of breastfeeding, and there are many studies including the Dundee Infant Feeding study which reported, in 1993, on the effects of early introduction of complementary foods on gastrointestinal illness. This report stated:

"The incidence was not related to the age of starting solid food with or without adjustment for the confounding variables of maternal age, social class, and type of milk feed. This suggests that, although there may be theoretical reasons

65

for infants not being able to tolerate solids in the first few months of life, in practice there is no significant gastrointestinal upset ... In our previous report on this cohort, breastfeeding for at least 13 weeks resulted in a significant reduction in episodes of gastrointestinal illness during the first year of life. This low incidence of gastrointestinal illness was seen in both the exclusively breastfed and the partially breastfed groups of infants, 65% of the second group having received solids before 13 weeks of age. The data from our two reports support the view that early introduction of solids does not increase the risk of gastrointestinal illness in infants, but continuation of breastfeeding is the key protective factor".

WHO STATEMENT 3

"The EFSA panel did not consider a large-group randomized trial in Belarus that is quite relevant to this issue. This trial found a 40% reduction in the odds of gastrointestinal infection in the arm with longer exclusive breastfeeding."

Author's comments: This statement references the PROBIT study (which is considered in detail in Chapter 8), and it is interesting because WHO were initially very focused on this study as their breastfeeding promotion programme was the intervention used to increase the duration of breastfeeding (and it was very effective). Moreover, the early data on the reduction of gastrointestinal illness in the longer-duration breastfeeding group was widely reported by WHO. However, the cohort has now been assessed for many other important health outcomes, at ages 6.5 years, 11.5 years and 16 years. The data at these later assessments indicate no additional benefit in the prolonged breastfeeding group, including effects on gastrointestinal illness. However, there is concern that at the age of 16 years the prolonged breastfeeding group showed evidence of increased overweight/obesity. The WHO have remained silent on these later findings.

WHO STATEMENT 4

"The WHA promotes exclusive breastfeeding for six months 'as a global public health recommendation'. The expert consultation that made this recommendation clarified that it applies to populations, acknowledging that individual infants may need to receive complementary foods before or after this exact age. The point of having public health recommendations is to provide general protection to the overall population while acknowledging individual variations."

Author's comments: Interestingly, the WHO are acknowledging that public health policies provide general protection to the overall population, and that individual infants may need complementary foods before or after six months of age. However, this small degree of flexibility in relation to policy has yet to be conceded in relation to *exclusive* breastfeeding – logic would dictate that flexibility in the timing of complementary feeding also requires flexibility in the timing of exclusive breastfeeding.

WHO STATEMENT 5

"The publication of the Panel's findings should include the interests declared by the authors regarding receipt of individual support from the food industry – both direct (e.g. consultancies, honoraria or travel support) and indirect (e.g. research grants). In addition, the source of funding for the work of the Panel is not clear. Given the commercial implications of the recommendations being made, this clarity is critical."

Author's comments: Declaration of interest is important, but it needs to apply to *all* organizations and should not only include financial interests but also all non-financial self-interests, including being a member of an organization that has a policy of non-cooperation with another partner organization. EFSA have the strictest policies and protocols on competing-interest management, and the attempt by WHO to undermine the governance standards of EFSA is surprising. Reference for the EFSA policy on competing interest is provided [8]

Casting aspersions aside, the academics and clinicians from across Europe (in addition to their normal day job) reviewed over three hundred publications to prepare this extensive document. Despite meeting the governance standards set by EFSA, WHO (surprisingly) thought it was appropriate to question their integrity – without producing any material evidence to support their comments. If WHO wished to see more information on the competing interests of the scientific and clinical contributors (in addition to that which was provided with the publication) they could have contacted EFSA directly. However, they clearly preferred to collude with their colleagues in breastfeeding activist groups rather than protect the scientists and clinicians who undertook the research for EFSA. In my opinion, this raises further questions about the professionalism, leadership and integrity of those who are in a position to influence infant-feeding policy. It is self-evident that WHO should be focusing on creating a unified stakeholder partnership, building on trust and respect.

Interestingly, WHO established a guideline development group in 2019 on complementary feeding of infants and children, which stated that:

"… *through its unique normative function in health, WHO aims to provide updated global guidance on complementary feeding of infants and children to promote optimal growth and development".*[9]

The expected outcome of the initial meeting was to have a consensus on a proposed outline for the guideline and the specific questions to be addressed. Not surprisingly, the membership of the guideline group includes WHO representatives, two senior figures from IBFAN and scientists with strong breastfeeding interests, but no authors of recent systematic reviews of complementary feeding or members from the infant food industry.

It is noted that even in the planning and development of policy for complementary feeding, WHO prefer to have the company of breastfeeding activist groups, rather than researchers and healthcare professionals who have made significant contributions to our understanding of the research and clinical need for complementary foods for infants and young children. The apparent collaborative research and educational activities with industry are viewed by WHO as deserving total exclusion from policy development. The purpose of this initial meeting on complementary feeding led by WHO was to obtain a 'consensus' on a proposed outline for the guideline on complementary feeding and to identify the specific questions to be addressed. However, it is obvious that if key stakeholders are excluded at this initial stage, then the views from the planning consensus are most likely to differ from the views of those who are excluded; therefore the expectation of consensus at the stage of delivery of the policy is unlikely. This inevitably leads to non-compliance, more conflict and again raises concerns about the quality of leadership.

Exclusive breastfeeding and the complementary feeding interface

To resolve the issues around the exclusive breastfeeding and complementary feeding interface, the evidence of underlying biological variation strongly supports the need for policy flexibility. For that reason, choosing an age range of four to six months to tentatively introduce complementary foods, would meet the needs of most infants. Infants themselves send a message that they are ready when they pick up a soft piece of fruit or vegetable, place it in their mouth, form a bolus and swallow – and subsequently look pleased at achieving a new developmental milestone. Alternatively, an infant may show no interest in solid foods before they are six months, which demonstrates the variation in normal human development. To highlight the importance of the relationship between the timing of introducing foods and the different milestones in infant development, note that infants from the age of six months begin learning how to close their mouths and turn their heads to refuse food. Thus the exposure to new tastes and textures before this time may benefit the establishment of a diverse solid-food diet. For this reason it is suggested that infant-feeding policies need to be cognizant with potential variations in feeding-related cognitive behaviours.

Cognitive behavioural aspects include 'responsive' feeding – a reciprocal relationship between an infant or child and their caregiver, characterized by the child communicating feelings of hunger and satiety through verbal or nonverbal cues, followed by an immediate response from the caregiver.[10] The response includes the provision of appropriate and nutritious food in a supportive manner, while maintaining an appropriate feeding environment. It is important for parents and health professionals to be familiar with responsive feeding, and aware of the possible 'cues' that can be exchanged between infants and caregivers. This can be considered as a 'conversation', conducted using sign language.

It has been suggested that responsive feeding is the foundation for the development of healthy eating behaviour, including self-regulation and self-control of food intake. Non-responsive feeding practices are reported to be associated with feeding problems and the development of under- or overnutrition.[10] As understanding of these interactions between infant and caregivers increases, the need for responsive infant-feeding policies that align with responsive feeding behaviours are required.

An integrated approach to infant and young-child feeding is essential

It is essential for complementary feeding to move out of the shadow of breastfeeding, and policy-makers need to focus on the complementary period during which the infant transitions from a liquid diet to a diverse family diet – a process that can have a significant impact on their future diet, health and life expectancy.

An analysis of nine resolutions relating to infant feeding issued by the WHA from 2005 to 2018 indicated that the word 'breastfeeding' was mentioned forty-one times, while the phrase 'complementary feeding' appeared only seven times. The WHO Strategy for Infant and Young-Child Feeding refers to breastfeeding seventy-three times and to complementary just twenty times. How much of this neglect of complementary feeding by policy-makers reflects the lack of interest groups to support complementary feeding?

There is a Global Breastfeeding Collective that currently involves at least twenty-five breastfeeding organizations. It is led by UNICEF and WHO.[11] Their mission is to rally political, legal, financial and public support, so that rates of breastfeeding increase, which will benefit mothers, children and society as a whole. There are *no* organizations that provide an equivalent level of support for complementary feeding. Why do these organizations distinguish between breastfeeding and complementary feeding when infants from the age of six months are dependent on both sources of nutrition to provide a balanced and nutritious diet?

This political separation between breastmilk and complementary foods is not only counterproductive in terms of partnership-working, but is a major contributor to the ongoing failure to improve the diet and nutritional status of children worldwide. With the recent report that the 'unintended consequences' of previous nutritional interventions may have contributed to the increasing prevalence of the double burden of malnutrition – and the assertion that this is related to silo policy-making – it is vitally important from both professional and ethical perspectives that preferences and prejudices are set aside and the focus is on all aspects of infant and young-child nutrition, with the key objective of serving the nutrition and healthcare needs of all children.[12] A greater focus on the word 'diet', even in infancy, reinforces the importance of a child not only receiving a balance of essential nutrients but also receiving the benefits of obtaining this through a range of different foods. This is particularly important during the complementary feeding period, when a diversity of foods nutritionally complements dietary intake, and also enables a range of flavours to be experienced and learned. This should be considered as an important evolutionary step towards a healthy diet for adults and children.

At present, the scientific evidence tends to focus on potential health benefits relating to breastfeeding and less frequently on the health effects relating to complementary feeding. Whereas the potential early and late health benefits of a balanced diet of liquid and solid foods in early life has not received the research, clinical and policymaking priority that it deserves.

Complementary feeding and malnutrition

The WHO/UN Strategic Development Goal 2 aims to achieve 'zero hunger' by 2030.[13] The problem is, if recent trends continue, the number of people affected by hunger will surpass 840 million by 2030. Malnutrition (consisting of undernutrition, overweight and obesity, and micronutrient deficiencies) continues to afflict millions of women and children, particularly in low-income and middle-income countries. Evidence on the effectiveness of antenatal multiple micronutrient supplementation in reducing the risk of stillbirths, low birthweight and born small-for-gestational-age babies has strengthened. Similarly evidence continues to support the provision of supplementary food in food-insecure settings. This includes community-based approaches on the use of locally produced supplementary and therapeutic food to manage children with acute malnutrition. Preventative nutritional interventions are listed in Box 5.2.

Box 5.2: Preventative nutritional interventions in children with acute malnutrition

- Promotion of breastfeeding
- Appropriate complementary feeding
- Zinc supplementation
- Periconceptual folic acid supplementation or fortification
- Maternal balanced energy protein supplementation
- Maternal multiple micronutrient (MMN) supplementation
- Maternal calcium supplementation
- Vitamin A supplementation
- General management of moderate and severe acute malnutrition
- This wealth of research evidence needs to be translated into targeted strategic and delivery plans that are scientifically based, but also pragmatic and achievable.

For progress to be achieved in meeting the SDG (sustainable development goal) relating to end of hunger and to achieve food security and improved nutrition for in infants and young children, stakeholders need to recognize their obligations to the provision of adequate nutrition for all young children worldwide, and in particular to the many millions of children who are currently experiencing the physical and cognitive consequences of malnutrition.[13]

The strategic goal for reducing child malnutrition and the prevalence of stunting has been set,[13] but specialist knowledge and expertise needs to come together to enable these objectives to be achieved. The target population is diverse, therefore a one-size-fits-all policy will not address the scope of the problem. For safe and nutritious complementary foods to reach *all* children, especially those in greatest need, a multilayer strategy – that sets out specific early-life nutrition safety nets – needs to be agreed. This should be accomplished by accepting that what is best for an infant living in a European city may differ from a child living in sub-Saharan Africa.

The nutritional tools available include breastmilk, infant formula, local complementary foods and commercial products. The different infant-feeding scenarios must be considered, and the approach to the most appropriate diet for each one must be agreed. For example, in infants from high-income countries, the current WHO infant and young-child feeding policy should be considered. However, infants living in conditions without clean water or sanitation, no access to breastmilk and inadequate local complementary foods, there should be a safety net that includes options for ready-to-use formula and ready-to-use commercial complementary foods.

To address this difficult problem, the focus has been on ready-to-use foods, ranging from those that are prepared locally to those that are commercially produced by national and international food companies. There are two categories of ready to use products:

- ready-to-use therapeutic foods (RUTFs) for treating severe acute malnutrition (SAM)
- ready-to-use supplement foods (RUSFs) targeted at children with moderate acute malnutrition (MAM).

It is suggested that RUSFs function better than the existing cereal blends used in food-aid programmes for MAM. Food products for MAM are categorized by the World Food Programme as treatment or prevention (or both), and as lipid-based or non-lipid-based. Specialized food products for managing MAM in infants below six months of age are not available, given that exclusive breastfeeding is recommended for this group.

UNICEF has been supportive of ready-to-use foods, however, organizations such as IBFAN are less enthusiastic and are reluctant to support the scaling up of RUSFs, as they believe this is largely commercially driven, and there should be a greater emphasis on supporting families in developing countries to feed themselves and to be empowered and educated to do so successfully and sustainably.[14] IBFAN is concerned that:

> "… malnutrition prevention and treatment are becoming increasingly medicalized with the use of fortified commercial foods as 'quick fixes', ignoring community-based approaches and the underlying basic causative factors".

It points out that:

> "… meanwhile, breastfeeding and adequate complementary feeding continue to receive scant funding and attention despite the large body of research that demonstrates it is (by far) the most effective and sustainable intervention to positively impact child health and survival".[14]

The Lancet's *Maternal and Child Health Series* highlighted MAM management, as well as SAM management, as an evidence-based intervention of sufficiently proven efficacy to warrant action at scale. A key message was that treatment strategies for SAM with recommended packages of care and ready-to-use therapeutic foods are well established, but further evidence is needed for prevention and management strategies for MAM in population settings.[15]

The inclusion of a target for reducing wasting among the six nutrition WHA goals for 2030 brings a sharper focus to MAM and SAM.[13] Approaches tend to be product focused and do not always take into account the underlying causes of malnutrition, and factors such as housing, clean water and sanitation need to be simultaneously addressed, as the child, after nutritional management, returns to the conditions that caused the malnutrition in the first place.

The WHO position is described in a Technical Note published in 2012.[16] This states that the dietary management of children with MAM should be based on the optimal use of locally available foods to improve nutritional status and to prevent the condition from deteriorating to SAM. In situations of food shortage or inadequate availability of some nutrients through local foods, supplementary foods can be used to treat children with MAM. However, the WHO 2012 Technical Note concludes:

> "… there are no evidence-informed recommendations on the composition of supplementary foods used to treat children with moderate acute malnutrition".[16]

With several millions of children dying each year from the effects of malnutrition, the WHO response is disappointing and gives an impression of a lack of urgency which continued over the subsequent years. However, in November 2019, seven years after the Technical Note, WHO announced that it proposes providing global, evidence-informed recommendations on the efficacy, safety and effectiveness of RUTFs for treating infants and children aged six months or older with uncomplicated SAM.[17] It will be interesting to see whether industry are considered to have a role in this initiative and – most importantly – whether those involved can generate the much-needed impetus to bring forward effective recommendations that will lead to actions capable of saving the lives of these vulnerable children. A paragraph in *The Lancet* series on malnutrition may provide a relevant perspective:[15]

> "The scale, know-how, reach, financial resources and existing involvement of the private sector in actions that affect nutrition status is well known. Yet there are still too few independent and rigorous assessments of the effectiveness of involvement of the commercial sector in nutrition. Distrust of the private sector – especially

the food industry – remains high and is linked, partly, to the decades-long tussle related to the marketing of breastmilk substitutes in developing countries and around continued marketing of sugar-sweetened beverages and fast foods worldwide. This troubled history has made it more difficult for the private sector to be a major contributor to the collective creation and sustenance of momentum for reduction of malnutrition. In view of the needs and substantial resources, influence, and convening power of the private sector, it might represent a missed opportunity. Opportunities exist for collaboration around advocacy, monitoring, value chains, technical and scientific collaboration, and staple-food fortification that are uncontentious and deserve further exploration. Knowledge in this area must be expanded rapidly to guide the private sector toward more positive effects for nutrition. Regulatory and fiscal efforts are essential when the private sector is involved in marketing of products that are detrimental to optimum nutrition. The experience gained with the International Code of Marketing of Breastmilk Substitutes should be applied to the promotion of other harmful, widely-consumed food products that are being marketed for young children".

This statement encapsulates how we should proceed with infant and young-child feeding. It identifies the opportunities for partnership-working with the food industry, it acknowledges the history, and recognizes the risks and the need for appropriate regulation to guide the private sector towards a more responsible and effective contribution to the infant and young-child diet. And finally, the lessons learned from the Code for breastmilk substitutes – good and bad – can be applied to any food products that are marketed for young children.

References

1. WHO (1998) *Complementary feeding of young children in developing countries: a review of current scientific knowledge.* Available at: https://apps.who.int/iris/handle/10665/65932 (last accessed August 2022).

2. WHO/UNICEF (2002) *Global strategy for infant and young child feeding.* Available at: http://apps.who.int/iris/bitstream/10665/42590/1/9241562218.pdf?ua=1&ua=1 (last accessed August 2022).

3. PAHO (2003) *Guiding principles for complementary feeding of the breastfed child.* Available at: http://www.who.int/nutrition/publications/guiding_principles_compfeeding_breastfed.pdf (last accessed August 2022).

4. WHO (2005) *Guiding principles for feeding non-breastfed children 6–24 months of age.* Available at: https://www.who.int/news/item/15-01-2011-exclusive-breastfeeding-for-six-months-best-for-babies-everywhere (last accessed February 2022).

4. WHO (2005) *Guiding principles for feeding non-breastfed children 6–24 months of age.* Available at: https://www.who.int/news/item/15-01-2011-exclusive-breastfeeding-for-six-months-best-for-babies-everywhere (last accessed February 2022).

5. UNICEF (2016) *From the first sign of life.* Available at: https://www.unicef.org/media/49801/file/From-the-first-hour-of-life-ENG.pdf (last accessed February 2022).

6. Castenmiller J, de Henauw S, Hirsch-Ernst K, *et al.* (European Food Safety Authority NDA Panel) (2019) Scientific Opinion on the appropriate age range for introduction of complementary feeding into an infant's diet. *EFSA Journal* 17, 5780.

7. Baby Milk Action (2019) *EFSA's faulty consultation on the age of introduction of baby foods closes.* Available at: http://www.babymilkaction.org/archives/21087 (accessed August 2022).

8. European Food Safety Authority (2018) *EFSA rules on competing interest management.* Available at: https://www.efsa.europa.eu/sites/default/files/corporate_publications/files/competing_interest_management_17.pdf (last accessed August 2022).

9. WHO (2019) *WHO Guideline Development Group. Meeting on complementary feeding of infants and children.* Available at: https://www.who.int/news-room/events/detail/2019/12/02/default-calendar/who-guideline-development-group-meeting-on-complementary-feeding-of-infants-and-children (last accessed February 2022).

10. Harbron J, Booley S, Najaar B, Day CE (2013) Responsive feeding: establishing healthy eating behaviour early on in life. *South African Journal of Clinical Nutrition* 26 (*Suppl.*) S141–49.

11. WHO/UNICEF (2017) *Global Breastfeeding Collective.* Available at: https://www.globalbreastfeedingcollective.org/ (last accessed February 2022).

12. Branca F, Demaio A, Udomkesmalee E *et al.* (2020) A new nutrition manifesto for a new nutrition reality. *The Lancet* 395, 8–10.

13. WHO (2015) *Sustainable Development Goals for 2030.* Available at: https://www.who.int/health-topics/sustainable-development-goals#tab=tab_1 (last accessed August 2022).

14. IBFAN (2014) *The advantages, disadvantages and risks of ready-to-use foods. Breastfeeding Briefs No. 56/57.* Available at: http://ibfan.org/breastfeedingbreafs/BB%2056-57-The%20advantages-disadvantages-and-risks-of-ready-to-use%20foods.pdf (last accessed August 2022).

15. Maternal and Child Health Study Group (2013) *Maternal and Child Nutrition Series. Executive Summary of The Lancet Maternal and Child Nutrition Series.* Available at: https://www.thelancet.com/pb/assets/raw/Lancet/stories/series/nutrition -eng.pdf (last accessed August 2022).

16. WHO (2012) *Supplementary foods for the management of moderate acute malnutrition in infants and children 6–59 months of age. Technical note.* Available at: https://apps.who.int/iris/handle/10665/75836 (last accessed August 2022).

17. WHO Guideline Development Group (2019) *The efficacy, safety and effectiveness of ready-to-use therapeutic foods (RUTF).* Available at: https://www.who.int/docs/default-source/blue-print/call-for-comments/2019-gdgmeeting-guideline-rutf-reduced-milkprotein-7nov-scopeandpurpose.pdf?sfvrsn=2a96a2d4_5 (last accessed August 2022).

CHAPTER 6

Is non-compliance prevalent across all stakeholders?

The infant-formula industry is widely considered to be the *bête noire* within the infant-feeding community, with frequent claims that they adopt marketing and sales practices that are not compliant with the Code.[1] Furthermore, it is argued that the infant-formula industry is primarily responsible for static or decreasing breastfeeding rates across the developing and developed world. This has generated decades of conflict that has led to high-profile boycotts and legal actions. More recently it has been claimed that the industry's behaviour is counter to human and planetary health.[2]

The response from the WHO has been to place further restrictions on the activities of industry through a series of additional WHA resolutions. Despite these measures, however, non-compliance, conflict and hostility prevail.

Although the marketing activities of the formula industry were the driving force for the introduction of the Code, the document includes many recommendations that relate to other stakeholders including governments, health services and parents.[3,4] This is a reflection of the multi-stakeholder system required to deliver optimum nutrition to infants worldwide, which needs to be driven by evidence-based policies, effective implementation systems, and governance structures that are proportionate and robust. But it is also important that the whole process engenders a sense of ownership and inclusiveness, in particular to make sure that consumers are able to comprehend how evidence and policy relate to them as individuals. Systemic deficiency at any point in this multilayer process may not only increase the risk of non-compliance by the infant-formula industry, but also reflect non-compliance with the Code by the other key stakeholders.

Note also that the articles contained within the Code refer to the health service, to health professionals, to industry and to parents, but none relate to the role of policy-makers or breastfeeding advocates and activists.

Evidence of lack of commitment to the Code by governments

A key decision by the WHA when endorsing the Code was that it should be adopted as a *recommendation*, rather than a *regulation*, and that the implementation of the Code should be closely monitored according to existing WHO constitutional procedures.[1] The Code is monitored through the WHO national member states, who are required to communicate annually to the Director-General with information on actions taken to give effect to the principles and aim of the Code. In even-numbered years the Director-General reports to the WHA on the status of implementation of the Code.

The reality is that compliance with this monitoring process is poor. In 2010, three decades after the Code's publication, WHO reported to the 63rd WHA on Infant and Child Nutrition that only ninety-two out of a hundred and ninety-three member states (just 48%) responded to the annual request by the WHO Secretariat for an update on progress prior to the forthcoming Assembly.[5] In response to the report to the WHA, the Code Secretariat identified several areas for action, including advocacy, operational research, training and monitoring, and they stated that actions will be initiated in the biennium (2010–2011) 'subject to sufficient funding'.

When the Code was published, the WHA 'urged' all member states to give full and unanimous support to the implementation of the Code. However, this approach of shared understanding and commitment has clearly not been successful. Raising an arm in support of a proposed action at a WHA annual meeting is a simple act but being faced with implementation at a local level is proving to be far more complex.

In 2011, the report from IBFAN, entitled the *State of the Code by Country*, confirmed that even in the member states that adopted the Code the measures taken are variable and limited. Their findings were that only sixty-seven of the one hundred and ninety-three member states (only 34.7%) had enacted legislation or adopted regulations, decrees or other legally binding measures that encompass provisions of the Code and subsequent WHA resolutions. Furthermore, forty-three of them (22.3%) had no active measures in place. In the remaining eighty-three (43.0%), the status varied from a few provisions in law to different levels of voluntary provision. In 2016, 135 countries had some form of Code-related legal measures in place, an increase from 103 in 2011. However, only 39 countries have legislation incorporating all or most Code provisions.[5]

From April 2020, data collection has been led by WHO in partnership with UNICEF and IBFAN, and current data suggest that 136 (70%) of a hundred and ninety-four WHO member states had enacted some legal measures with provisions to implement the Code.[6] However, of these, not one country was fully aligned with the Code; only twenty-five countries (12.8%) had measures that were substantially aligned with the Code. A further forty-two had measures that are moderately aligned. Sixty-nine had some provisions, and fifty-eight had no legal provisions. There is a clear separation between developing countries, in which the legal provisions are most prevalent, and developed countries in which implementation is minimal.

The primary objective of the Code was to prevent inappropriate marketing and promotion of breastmilk substitutes and, in so doing, protect breastfeeding. So this is primarily an industry matter and is specifically related to trading standards. However, the recommendations within the Code place restrictions on healthcare workers and parents, and the expectation by WHO – that governments should legislate against doctors, midwives, community nurses and parents to try and mitigate the behaviour of industry – will undoubtedly contribute to the low implementation rates.

Legislation should be targeted *directly* at the infant-formula industry, and *precisely* at the standards required for placing a product on the market. This should include all material relating to the marketing and promotion of the product. Currently infant formula products and related marketing material can be launched into the market without pre-market scrutiny by an independent regulatory body. This is discussed more fully in Chapter 14, in which the option of a global trading standards office with a primary focus on breastmilk substitutes is considered.

Evidence of failure of compliance by health services

The recommended role that health services and healthcare workers have in promoting and protecting breastfeeding is highlighted in Articles 6 and 7 of the Code,[2] which set out specific conditions regarding their relationship with industry, including:

- the exchange of information with manufacturers
- potential financial inducements from industry
- receipt of samples and equipment
- financial support for research and education.

However, as mentioned later in Chapter 10, it is also important that the interface between the health professional and the parent (so critical during a child's early life) is not fractured by legislative interventions that could be viewed as interfering with normal clinical practice.

It is understood that systems must be in place that ensure contact between healthcare workers and industry does not undermine support for breastfeeding, although it is noted that women are far more likely to cease breastfeeding because of basic preventable healthcare issues such as painful breasts, concerns about the adequacy of their milk supply, and a perception that the infant is not satiated. It is therefore important that healthcare services are designed to provide quality care to mothers and their infants, and systems are in place to assure governments that clinical practice meets agreed standards.

The Baby Friendly Initiative (BFI) was launched in 1991 with the objective of providing a global approach to the monitoring of maternity services and, in particular, to ensure breastfeeding is supported in accordance with the Code. In 1998, its principles were extended to cover the work of community healthcare services with the *Seven Point Plan for the Promotion, Protection and Support of Breastfeeding in Community Health Care Settings.*[7]

Despite universal recognition of the benefits of breastfeeding – and claims that BFI accreditation improves breastfeeding outcomes – global implementation has been slow, particularly in high-income countries. Numerous obstacles to and constraints on implementation have been identified. These include the need for:

- additional resources for BFI implementation
- more effective leadership of practice change
- training healthcare workers to improve breastfeeding practices.

The adverse marketing activities by infant-formula companies were also noted, especially by breastfeeding activist groups. These findings of disappointing progress are consistent with UNICEF's 2005 review of the Innocenti Declaration, which identified that the main challenges to BFI implementation were the commitment of staff, the associated financial costs, and the importance of a continuum of care across the community.[7,8] However, more recent reviews of the BFI have raised issues of:

- unrealistic expectations of breastfeeding
- not meeting women's individual needs
- fostering negative emotional experiences.

These were discussed in Chapter 4.

Although costs and service structures are clearly important, the success of breastfeeding depends heavily upon a shared understanding and commitment from both healthcare staff and the mothers they are supporting. For this to be assured, staff and mothers should not feel pressure to adopt practices that they do not feel serve the interests of a particular infant and family. The key messages – that the infant should initially receive exclusive breastmilk, followed by the introduction of solid foods, then gradually transition to a nutritious family diet – are fully understood. The areas of discussion and potential vulnerability of the process are the *timings* that are dictated by WHO for the transition periods:

- exclusive breastfeeding for six months
- continued breastfeeding for two years or beyond
- complementary feeding at six months
- any milk product marketed for children up to three years 'should be understood' to be a breastmilk substitute.

The issue is that health professionals and parents have difficulty with the assumption that this inflexibility can be applied to all infants worldwide, and this is a constant source of questions and heated discussion. Moreover, from a health professional perspective the ethical concern is that clinical judgement may be viewed by others as a violation of the Code.

It is unfortunate that the Code was written *by* bureaucrats *for* bureaucrats, as this has excluded what is most important for successful breastfeeding – namely, empathy. The inability of policymakers to accept that infants are individuals and that there is a range of normality, is considered by parents as a major contributor to the emotions and anxiety mothers can feel when breastfeeding. For those stakeholders who are more closely involved in delivering healthcare support, policies that not only acknowledge and address the emotional needs of parents but are written in a language that reflects the need for each infant to be accepted as an individual, would be more receptive.

This requires messages to be more implicit, using qualifier terms such as 'perhaps', 'possibly' and 'maybe' – words that acknowledge the inevitable variation and thus reduce levels of reactance. However, language that is 'controlling' includes forceful adverbs such as 'ought', 'must' and 'should'.[9] It is noted that in the WHO Code, the word 'should' appears ninety-six times, but the words 'perhaps', 'possibly' and 'maybe' are not used at all.

The confidence of parents and health professionals is critical for a successful breastfeeding experience. A key element underpinning this confidence is that there is a safety net, in the form of infant formula. In other settings, the presence of a safety net enables individuals to try things they may not otherwise try. In the discourses on infant-formula companies, it is important to separate the importance of having infant formulas as a safety net (which can reduce morbidity and mortality in the absence of breastmilk) from the unprofessional marketing and sales activities of the companies. This point is clearly stated in the Code:

> *"Considering that, when mothers do not breastfeed, or only do so partially, there is a legitimate market for infant formula and for suitable ingredients from which to prepare it; that all these products should accordingly be made accessible to those who need them through commercial or non-commercial distribution systems; and that they should not be marketed or distributed in ways that may interfere with the protection and promotion of breastfeeding".*

Evidence of failure to govern the Code

Proposals regarding the monitoring of the implementation of the Code are included in Article 11. It is noted that manufacturers and distributors of products within the scope of the Code should, independently of any other measures taken for its implementation, regard themselves as responsible for monitoring their marketing practices according to the principles and aim of the Code. Article 11 also states that NGOs, professional groups, institutions and individuals should have the responsibility of drawing the attention of manufacturers or distributors to activities that are incompatible with the Code, and the appropriate governmental authority should also be informed.

A self-regulatory structure for such a disparate group of organizations is unlikely to succeed, and an overall regulatory system is required. The option of an 'ombudsman', or an independent governance body with the authority to arbitrate and ensure that actions taken by respective parties are in keeping with the spirit of the Code, has been suggested.[3] Such a governance body would need to have jurisdiction over all stakeholders, including WHO and WHA. The Code was written and endorsed by WHO and WHA, and there appears to be an assumption that they can modify the meaning of some aspects of it through 'subsequent resolutions', without having formal discussions with the wider stakeholder community. Thus, from a governance perspective, clarification is required on whether this is within their right, and whether it is an appropriate line of action in relation to governance standards. An independent review would certainly focus on the governance arrangements. This is considered further in Chapter 16.

The non-cooperation between WHO and industry has led to two separate approaches to Code governance. The WHO established a monitoring system called NetCode in partnership with UN system organizations, WHO Collaborating Centres, NGOs that are particularly active in supporting breastfeeding, and selected WHO member states.[10] Their key objective is to monitor compliance with the Code and to:

> *"… hold manufacturers, distributors, retail outlets, the healthcare system and healthcare workers to account for their breaches of national laws and/or the Code".*

NetCode is not independent and it is clearly divisive, with one half of the infant-feeding community monitoring the other half. Note that this is not a reciprocal arrangement and this will be discussed further in Chapter 14.

An unexpected but interesting initiative addressing governance of infant-formula manufacturers has now emerged. The initiative is led by the FTSE Group, which is an independent company jointly owned by the *Financial Times* and the London Stock Exchange Group – a world leader in the development of indices used by investors to assess business portfolios, performance and risks. In 2001, FTSE launched 'FTSE4Good', which was designed to act as a tool for investors who are interested in companies with acknowledged records of corporate social responsibility, including environmental sustainability, human rights and stakeholder involvement. Following discussions with UNICEF, FTSE4Good has established an index for companies that operate in the breastmilk substitute sector. The expectation is that these companies will secure their inclusion in the FTSE4Good investment index by demonstrating that they meet specific marketing standards.[11] This initiative, and a more recent audit organization – the *Access to Nutrition Index* – are discussed in more detail in Chapter 14.

Non-compliance issues for families

Policy and codes of practice have to adapt to societal change. For example, there has been a rapid expansion of the female workforce, but how do current infant-feeding policies, and the Code, impact on working mothers and the welfare needs of their families? From a government perspective, the potential cost of additional maternity leave must be related to the strength of evidence on additional health gain. Moreover, Article 4 of the Code makes specific recommendations on information and education and, in particular, the limits within which formula companies can disseminate information on their products.

The general public today expect to have immediate access to electronically delivered information. They are accustomed to the process of assimilating information and making choices. It is extremely important for parents to be provided with the most up-to-date information on infant feeding, with a transparent and balanced approach regarding both breastmilk and infant formula. Concern has already been expressed that internet social networking may be an increasing area of non-compliance by infant-formula companies, so there are pleas for tighter controls. The level of control should be carefully considered, of course, because it is important to respect the right of parents to seek information from different sources and to develop a feeding plan that they believe is best for their baby, and which reflects their social and economic circumstances.

Societies in all countries worldwide have changed in the last forty years, and the Code is older than most new mothers today. The assertion that the Code does not need to be reviewed or updated is difficult to justify and will continue to be a source of discontent. It is important that the current generation of parents have an opportunity to contribute to a document that dictates so many aspects of infant feeding and is the source of so much debate and discord. Moreover, it is not only new mothers who have not had an opportunity to provide a contemporary view on the Code, as this situation also applies to health professionals, policymakers and even industry representatives, and of course, those individuals who signed up to the Code in 1981 are unlikely to be in a position to be held accountable.

A way forward

Non-compliance with the WHO Code is evident at all levels of the implementation process and this systemic failure needs to be urgently addressed. To clarify the issues and identify solutions there needs to be effective participation and collaboration of all key stakeholders. However, because of the protracted period of acrimony and atmosphere of mistrust that has now become embedded between key agencies, to achieve effective partnership-working within an environment of trust, respect, shared understanding and governance, the development of a 'memorandum of understanding' (MoU) is proposed. This would set out the common understandings, express a convergence of will between the parties, and indicate an intended common line of action. To reach agreement on the MoU and then to advance discussions on key infant-feeding matters, a number of options may be considered (see Chapter 17).

1. It would be constructive to identify where there is general consensus, and this will include - breast feeding being the optimal method to feed babies from birth; exclusive breast feeding recommended for six months in low-income countries and communities; and that marketing practices of the infant formula industry need to be effectively regulated.

2. It is important to identify what is not working and this includes the lack of an effective working relationship between the WHO and industry, the reluctance of governments to implement the Code in its entirety; a lack of formal governance structures to identify issues and take appropriate action; and a lack of effective engagement and shared understanding with families.

3. The validity of the WHO Code and subsequent resolutions need to be evaluated to determine if they remain as relevant today as they did in 1981. Although there may be justification for some revision of the document, particularly in the areas of information and education, the key principles relating to supporting and protecting breast feeding and the need for regulation of marketing activities of infant formula companies, remain valid today. What is critical, however, is that in each country the Code should relate to an infant-feeding policy that is sensitive to the contemporary needs of local populations.

4. A proposal to establish an external governance body with appropriate knowledge, expertise should be considered. An international governance board (IGB) would have the remit to advise WHO and WHA, governments and NGOs on the establishment of governance structures and systems that will underpin the Code, and other related policies. The relationship with key stakeholders such as the WHO, will need to be determined and it is essential that the membership of the governance body has the confidence of all interested parties and that processes are informed, transparent and independent.

5. Governance structures specific for each of the stakeholders need to be strengthened. There should be an effective and sustainable governance system for monitoring compliance with the Code by the infant formula industry, and the potential options of using modern technology need to be considered (Chapter 14); moreover, governance needs to apply to WHO and WHA, especially as the latter is the global decision-making body for infant and child nutrition; governments and their healthcare systems need to establish transparent governance and reporting systems that provide robust and complete data on compliance with both the Code and infant-feeding policy; special interest groups need to ensure that their activities meet agreed governance standards; and finally, all governance related information should be available within the public domain.

Conclusion

Non-compliance with the WHO Code is not confined to the infant-formula industry. There is evidence of systemic failings at all levels of the implementation and monitoring process. Although all key stakeholders need to take responsibility for non-compliance with the WHO Code, and collectively address the most pressing issues, the primary focus is on the activities and behaviour of industry. A solution is required that does not have a negative impact on health professionals and parents.

A root-and-branch review, that was not sanctioned by WHO/WHA, has recently been undertaken on the Code and this should form the benchmark for change.[12] It is fundamentally important to clearly define the elements of evidence, policy, practice and governance for both developing and developed countries, and it may be beneficial to reflect on the vision of those who initiated the Code, and to concur that participation and cooperation are essential if global improvements in infant nutrition are to be achieved.

Addendum

This chapter is based on a previously published article: Forsyth JS (2013) Non-compliance with the International Code of Marketing of Breastmilk Substitutes is not confined to the infant-formula industry (2013) *Journal of Public Health* 35, 185–90. At the time of publication the Editor invited two commentaries on the article, which are summarized in Box 6.1 on the following pages.

> **Box 6.1: Summary of commentaries invited on the**
> **_Journal of Public Health_ article (2013)**
>
> **COMMENTARY 1—From BJ Hardy of the Ethical, Social and Cultural Program for Global Health, Sandra Rotman Centre, Toronto, Canada**
>
> Hardy's commentary noted that the Code remains an important yet deeply divisive piece of international policy intended to prevent inappropriate marketing and promote breastfeeding globally. It also acknowledged the argument that the Code had the opposite effect – it had driven a wedge between the various sectors needed to have dialogues and collaborate to promote breastfeeding.
>
> Hardy indicated that this criticism could be heard in the hallways at the 65th World Health Assembly in Geneva in May 2013, and was related to, more broadly, the general atmosphere of mistrust between stakeholders in the infant and young-child nutrition community.

Hardy reflected on the proposal of a MoU to be established between key agencies to set out common understandings, to express a convergence of will between parties, and to indicate an intended mutual line of action. She looked upon this favourably but emphasised the importance of identifying concrete steps that would be required to convince various actors from the public and private sectors to come together to discuss challenges and build trust. Helpfully, she made reference to a programme of a proposed set of shared principles of ethics for infants and young children in the developing world – derived from relevant existing laws, trade regimens, international codes and international goals – from which stakeholders may be able to begin a dialogue around establishing an operational framework for cooperation, collaboration and oversight.[a] She added that stakeholders should explore the possibility of a multi-stakeholder initiative, analogous to the Ethical Trading Initiative, which was established to address sweatshop violations in the international labour industry.[b]

She reiterated the need for effective leadership to initiate the process of building the level of trust necessary for implementation, and suggested that WHO, along with other key international agencies, could act as a neutral arbitrator to negotiate the terms of a MoU between stakeholders. This might incorporate conflict-of-interest guidelines and the underlying shared ethical principles for infant and young-child feeding, as well as pointing out that the negative impact of the lack of dialogue between stakeholders in this area, specifically over the Code, should not be underestimated.

Hardy's final point was that, despite the deep divisions and perceived ineffectiveness of the Code, some stakeholder groups still think it should be extended to include complementary foods in addition to breastmilk substitutes. However, she felt that such a move would exacerbate international efforts to tackle infant and young-child undernutrition.

Source of commentary: Hardy BJ (2013) Getting to compliance. Multisector dialogue, collaboration and the international code of marketing of breastmilk substitutes. *Journal of Public Health (Oxf)* 352, 191–92. DOI: 10.1093/pubmed/fdt025/. Available at: https://pubmed.ncbi.nlm.nih.gov/23543796/.

Sources cited in the commentary

[a]Singh JA, Daar AS, Singer PA (2010) Shared principles of ethics for infant and young-child nutrition in the developing world. *BMC Public Health* 10, 321.

[b]Singer PA, Ansett S, Sagoe-Moses I (2011) What could infant and young-child nutrition learn from sweatshops? *BMC Public Health* 11, 276.

COMMENTARY 2—From Yeong Joo Kean of the International Code Documentation Centre, Penang, Malaysia

Yeong set out the accepted criticisms of the behaviour of the infant-formula industry, particularly in relation to the inappropriate marketing and promotion of infant-formula products, and the impact this is having on breastfeeding rates. She agreed that some stakeholders failed as duty-bearers to protect the best interest of children but emphasized that when it comes to unethical marketing and the ensuing harm to infant and young-child health, the fault must lie solely with industry. She also noted how forward-looking companies recognize that compliance is the price of doing business, and they are developing governance, risk and compliance initiatives to ensure greater corporate accountability. She indicated that industry should not be looking for excuses or soft alternatives where Code commitments are concerned.

Yeong was highly critical of FTSE with their criteria introducing a false distinction between high-risk countries those with at least 10 per 1000 under-five mortality rate – that require an acknowledgement that the adoption and adherence to the Code is a minimum requirement – and the rest of the world, that don't. She argued strongly that this is contrary to the WHA's position. The International Code is global and applies to all countries because parents and infants in industrialized countries deserve the same level of protection from inappropriate and unethical marketing as those in developing ones. Reference was made to the potential for significant healthcare savings if breastfeeding rates are upscaled to recommended levels. Moreover, in terms of policy, she supported WHO's approach of 'one size fits all' and viewed this as a way of controlling the behaviours of industry. She also believed that my paper underestimated the progress made in implementing the Code up to 2013, identifying achievements at a country level where Code-based law is implemented, addressing issues of labelling and curtailing promotional practices.

Lastly, Yeong raised questions about my suggestion of an independent' international governance board (IGB) to advise governments and organizations about establishing governance structures and systems that underpin the Code. She noted that there did not appear to be any parallel system that the IGB could be modelled on, and she and her colleagues were looking for concrete suggestions and the suggestions were not just ideological, but also logical. She concluded that by 'independent', it was hoped I meant the IGB would be free of commercial influence.

Source of commentary:

Yeong JK (2014) Non-compliance with the *International Code of Marketing of Breastmilk Substitutes* is not confined to the infant-formula industry. *Public Health (Oxf)* 2014, 352, 193–94. DOI: 10.1093/pubmed/fdt026/. Available at: https://pubmed.ncbi.nlm.nih.gov/23564839/.

The two commentaries acknowledged that there are ongoing issues regarding the Code – in particular – with compliance, implementation and monitoring, but they offered differences in approach, especially in relation to the interface with industry. The issues identified within these commentaries are considered in more detail throughout this book. One important consideration is whether the committed direction of travel pursued by Yeong Joo Kean and her colleagues will ultimately lead to fulfilling their global vision of optimum infant feeding – or whether factors beyond the infant food industry, such as societal, cultural, health and economic change, will inevitably create new and alternative perspectives on how the nutritional needs of infants and young children can be met

References

1. WHO (1981) *International Code of Marketing of Breastmilk Substitutes.* Available at: https://apps.who.int/iris/bitstream/handle/10665/40382/9241541601.pdf?sequence=1&isAllowed=y (last accessed August 2022).

2. Branca F, Demaio A, Udomkesmalee E *et al.* (2020) A new nutrition manifesto for a new nutrition reality. *The Lancet* 395, 8–10.

3. Forsyth S (2010) *International Code of Marketing of Breastmilk Substitutes* – three decades later time for hostilities to be replaced by effective national and international governance. *Archives of Diseases in Childhood* 95, 769–70.

4. Forsyth S (2013) Non-compliance with the *International Code of Marketing of Breastmilk Substitutes* is not confined to the infant-formula industry. *Journal of Public Health* 35, 185–90.

5. WHO/UNICEF/IBFAN (2016) *Marketing of Breastmilk Substitutes: National Implementation of the International Code. Status Report 2016.* Available at: https://www.who.int/publications/i/item/9789241565325 (last accessed August 2022).

6. WHO/UNICEF/IBFAN (2020) *Marketing of Breastmilk Substitutes: National Implementation of the International Code. Status Report 2020.* Available at: https://www.who.int/publications/i/item/9789240006010 (last accessed August 2022).

7. UNICEF. *Baby Friendly Initiative*. Available at: https://www.unicef.org.uk/babyfriendly/ (last accessed August 2022).

8. Innocenti Declaration (2005) *On infant and young-child feeding*. Available at: http://www.unicef.org/programme/breastfeeding/innocenti.htm (last accessed August 2022).

9. Rosenberg BD, Siegel JT (2018) *Motivation Science* 4, 281–300.

10. WHO/UN Children's Fund (2017) *NetCode toolkit. Monitoring the marketing of breastmilk substitutes: protocol for ongoing monitoring systems*. Licence CC BY-NC-SA 3.0 IGO. Available at: https://apps.who.int/iris/handle/10665/259441 (last accessed August 2022).

11. Forsyth S (2012) FTSE, WHO Code and the infant-formula industry. *Annals of Nutrition and Metabolism* 60, 154–56. DOI: 10.1159/000337304.

12. Evans A (2018) *Food for thought. An independent assessment of the International Code of Marketing of Breastmilk Substitutes*. Breastfeeding Innovation Team. Available at: https://medium.com/@JustACTIONS/food-for-thought-an-independent-assessment-of-the-international-code-of-marketing-of-breast-milk-1d8d704ee612 (last accessed August 2022).

CHAPTER 7

When is a breastmilk substitute no longer a breastmilk substitute?

Infant-feeding policies should ensure that during the transition from exclusive breastfeeding to a family diet, infants and young children experience a continuum of key food sources that meet the energy and nutrition requirements for rapid growth and development.

During the first six months of life this can be achieved by exclusive breastfeeding, but beyond the age of six months there is a critical nutritional interdependence between breastmilk and complementary foods, which needs to evolve during the complementary feeding period.

Breastfeeding is the ideal for all newborn infants, yet – in practice – compliance can vary. Recognizing the right of every child to be adequately nourished, it was acknowledged in the Code that when mothers do not breastfeed, or only do so partially, there is a legitimate market for infant formulas.[1] The Code defines 'breastmilk substitutes' as:

> "… any food being marketed or otherwise presented as a partial or total replacement for breastmilk, whether or not suitable for that purpose".

However, in 2016 a document prepared by the WHO Secretariat for discussion at the 69th World Health Assembly titled *Guidance on Ending the Inappropriate Promotion of Foods for Infants and Young Children* stated under Recommendation 2 that:

> "… breastmilk substitute should be understood to include any milks (or products that could be used to replace milk, such as fortified soy milk), in either liquid or powdered form, that are specifically marketed for feeding infants and young children up to the age of 3 years (including follow-up formula and growing-up milks)".[2]

This statement by WHO is in conflict with the definition of breastmilk substitutes in the Code and it blurs the boundaries between breastmilk substitutes and complementary foods. This wording emerged without evidence of consultation with key stakeholders, and its policy status and scientific credibility needs to be carefully evaluated.

What is the policy status of this new interpretation of breastmilk substitutes?

The issue of inappropriate promotion of foods for infants and young children has been a longstanding concern and, in response to a request at the 65fth WHA in 2012 for the issue to be reviewed, the Department of Nutrition for Health and Development at WHO established the Scientific and Technical Advisory Group (STAG). This was in 2013.

The aim of STAG was to provide clarification on what constitutes 'inappropriate promotion' of foods for infants and young children.[3] It provided WHO with a report in 2015, which included several recommendations, emphasizing the importance of existing international instruments, particularly the scope of the Code as set out in Article 2, and clarifying key definitions. But it made no reference to changes in breastmilk substitute terminology or interpretation – that all milk products specifically marketed for feeding infants and young children up to the age of three years should be called breastmilk substitutes.

Subsequently, the document that WHO Secretariat prepared for the 69th WHA (69.7 Add.1) entitled *Guidance on Ending the Inappropriate Promotion of Foods for Infants and Young Children,* included their new interpretation of the term 'breastmilk substitute'.[2] There was no background information to explain this unexpected development.

The 69.7 Add.1 document was one of the accompanying reports for the discussion at the WHA (agenda item 12.1) on 28 May 2016. The subsequent official resolution document reporting on the outcome of the WHA discussion on this item (WHA 69.9) made no reference to a change in the definition or the interpretation of the term 'breastmilk substitute'.[4]

Since then, questions have been asked on the policy status of the Secretariat Guidance and, specifically, the origins of the three-year recommendation. It now appears that the proposal to include a three-year timeline for the term breastmilk substitutes was suggested in comments received by WHO from the Infant Feeding Action Coalition (INFACT) Canada and IBFAN.

This precipitated introduction of the new three-year timeline and the new definition of a breastmilk substitute now has limited resemblance to the original Code definition (Box 7.1).

Box 7.1: The evolving 'clarification' of the term 'breastmilk substitutes'

Original definition—WHO International Code of Marketing of Breastmilk Substitutes (May 1981)

"'Breastmilk substitute' means any food being marketed or otherwise presented as a partial or total replacement for breastmilk, whether or not suitable for that purpose."

First clarification—WHO Discussion Paper: Clarification and Guidance on Inappropriate Promotion of Foods for Infants and Young Children (20 July 2015)

"Implementation of the International Code of Marketing of Breastmilk Substitutes should clearly cover all products that function as breastmilk substitutes. This should include any milk products (liquid or powdered) marketed for young children up to **two years** [author's emphasis] including follow-up formula and growing-up milks)."

Second clarification—INFACT Canada/IBFAN Comment on the Discussion Paper: WHO Clarification and Guidance on Inappropriate Promotions of Foods for Infants and Young Children (20 July 2015)

"Implementation of the International Code of Marketing of Breastmilk Substitutes should clearly cover all products that function as breastmilk substitutes. This should include any milk products (liquid or powdered) marketed for young children up to **three years** [author's emphasis] (including follow-up formula and growing-up milks)".

Third clarification—Guidance on Ending the Inappropriate Promotion of Foods for Infants and Young Children. Report by the Secretariat, World Health Organization (WHA 69.7 Add.1, May 2016)

"A breast-milk substitute should be understood to include any milks (or products that could be used to replace milk, such as fortified soy milk), in either liquid or powdered form, that are specifically marketed for feeding infants and young children up to the age of **three years** [author's emphasis] (including follow-up formula and growing-up milks). It should be clear that the implementation of the International Code of Marketing of Breast-milk Substitutes and subsequent relevant Health Assembly resolutions covers all these products."

Is WHO's interpretation of breastmilk substitutes plausible?

In addition to questioning the due diligence of the policy-making process, it is important to examine the appropriateness of WHO interpretation. Annex 3 of the Code[1] contains excerpts from the Introductory Statement by the Representative of the Executive Board to the 34th WHA on the Subject of the Draft *International Code of Marketing of Breastmilk Substitutes*. Previous reference has been made to these statements, but because of their relevance to this issue it is worth re-stating the contribution of WHO Executive Board member, Dr Torbjørn Mork Director-General of Health Services, Norway:

> *"The scope of the draft code is defined in Article 2. During the first four to six months of life, breastmilk alone is usually adequate to sustain the normal infant's nutritional requirements. Breastmilk may be replaced (substituted for) during this period by bona fide breastmilk substitutes, including infant formula. Any other food, such as cow's milk, fruit juices, cereals, vegetables, or any other fluid, solid or semisolid food intended for infants and given after this initial period, can no longer be considered as a replacement for breastmilk (or as its bona fide substitute). Such foods only complement breastmilk or breastmilk substitutes and are thus referred to in the draft Code as complementary foods. They are also commonly called weaning foods or breastmilk supplements. Products other than bona fide breastmilk substitutes, including infant formula, are covered by the code only when they are 'marketed or otherwise represented to be suitable ... for use as a partial or total replacement of breastmilk. Thus the Code's references to products used as partial or total replacements for breastmilk are not intended to apply to complementary foods unless these foods are actually marketed as being suitable for the partial or total replacement of breastmilk. So long as the manufacturers and distributors of the products do not promote them as being suitable for use as partial or total replacements for breastmilk, then the Code's provisions concerning limitations on advertising and other promotional activities do not apply to these products".*

Moreover, it was further noted by Mork that:

> *"Several Executive Board members indicated that they considered introducing amendments in order to strengthen it and to make it still more precise. The Board considered, however, that the adoption of the Code by the Thirty-fourth World Health Assembly was a matter of great urgency in view of the serious situation prevailing, particularly in developing countries, and that amendments introduced*

at the present stage might lead to a postponement of the adoption of the Code. The Board therefore unanimously recommended to this Thirty-fourth World Health Assembly the adoption of the Code as presently drafted, realizing that it might be desirable or even necessary to revise the Code at an early date in the light of the experience obtained in the implementation of its various provisions. This is reflected in operative paragraph 5(4) of the recommended resolution contained in resolution EB67.R12".

This text provides an important insight into the thinking behind the Code at that time, and it is evident that the term 'breastmilk substitute' was focused on the first six months of life. This contrasts markedly with the statement from WHO in 2016, that the term applies to *all* milk products marketed for children up to the age of three years. This is allegedly a 'clarification' of the original Code definition, and not a redefining or reinterpretation.[5] However, this is difficult to comprehend and this point is not effectively addressed in WHO correspondence in the *Addendum* to this chapter. Also note that Annex 3 gives an indication that some revision of the Code may be required subsequently:

"... it might be desirable or even necessary to revise the code at an early date in the light of the experience obtained in the implementation of its various provisions".

Unfortunately this has not been formally initiated by WHO or WHA during the last forty years. It is quite obvious from these early understandings of the concept of a 'breastmilk substitute' that deciding whether a product replaces breastmilk or complements breastmilk is the *key* to whether a product is a breastmilk substitute or not. In the Code, infant formula is defined as a:

"... breastmilk substitute as it is designed to satisfy the normal nutritional requirements of infants up to and between four and six months of age, and in this role, it is replacing breastmilk".[1]

And complementary food is defined as:

"... any food, whether manufactured or locally prepared, that is suitable as a complement to breastmilk or to infant formula, when either may become insufficient to satisfy the nutritional requirements of the infant".

From these clear and logical definitions,[1] it can be concluded that complementary foods are *not* breastmilk substitutes, unless they are specifically marketed as providing partial or total replacement of breastmilk. However, the new WHO interpretation refers to:

"... any milks (or products that could be used to replace milk, such as fortified soy milk), in either liquid or powdered form, that are specifically marketed for feeding infants and young children up to the age of 3 years".[5]

The confusion may be reduced if it is understood that there is a difference between products that are marketed as suitable for children and those that are specifically marketed as a *replacement* for breastmilk. To be marketed as a replacement, the composition of the product must reflect the composition of breastmilk; whereas a product that is marketed as a complementary drink or food must reflect the nutritional requirements of a child during the complementary feeding period.

The age of three years has not previously been linked with the term 'breastmilk substitute'. In support of this age requirement, WHO referenced the Codex Alimentarius guidelines on formulated complementary foods for older infants and young children.[6] On examination of this document, the introduction provides several definitions, including a definition of 'young children' as persons from the age of more than twelve months up to the age of three years. However, the purpose of this document is to provide guidance on formulated complementary foods, which are described as:

> "... foods specifically formulated with appropriate nutritional quality to provide additional energy and nutrients to complement the family foods".

There was no suggestion that any of the guidance from that document relates to breastmilk substitutes, as confirmed in the final line of the document:

> "The products covered by these guidelines are not breastmilk substitutes and shall not be presented as such".

It is therefore concluded that the three-year age limit in the new breastmilk substitute interpretation lacks policy precedence. In 2001, when WHO considered whether follow-up formula is a 'breastmilk substitute' or not, it was commented:

> "... on the assumption that follow-up formula is not marketed or otherwise represented to be suitable as a breastmilk substitute, strictly speaking it does not fall within the scope of the International Code".[7]

More recently, WHO wording has been:

> "... follow-on milks (or follow-up formula) and growing-up milks are covered by the scope of the International Code. These milks function as de facto breastmilk substitutes because their consumption displaces rather than complements the intake of breastmilk. While they are compositionally different from infant formula, they partially or totally replace the consumption of breastmilk and as such should be considered to be breastmilk substitutes".[8]

There comes a time in these types of discussions where the reluctance to compromise results in an outcome that satisfies nobody and produces a contrived outcome that is a greater risk than the original issue. The failure to bring clarity to the above confusion is encapsulated in the statements in Table 7.1, which reflect statements included in the *Implementation Manual for Guidance on Ending the Inappropriate Promotion of Foods for Infants and Young Children.*[8]

Table 7.1: Confusion over breastmilk substitutes— statements from the *Implementation Manual for Guidance on Ending the Inappropriate Promotion of Foods for Infants and Young Children.*[8]

Are breastmilk substitutes	Are not breastmilk substitutes
A breastmilk substitute should be understood to include any milks (or products that could be used to replace milk, such as fortified soy milk), in either liquid or powdered form, that is specifically marketed for feeding infants and young children up to the age of three years (including follow-up formula and growing-up milks). It should be clear that the implementation of the Code and subsequent relevant resolutions cover all these products.	Milk products such as fresh or dried animal milks, fermented milk products, yoghurt or non-dairy milk alternatives are not covered by the Code and the 2016 Guidance as long as they are not labelled or marketed specifically for feeding infants and young children under thirty-six months. However, if they are marketed for this age range, they should not be treated differently from infant formula, follow-up formula or growing up milks, and as such fall within the scope of the Code and are subject to the recommendations set forth in the Guidance.
Products that function as breastmilk substitutes should not be promoted, because this may interfere with breastfeeding.	Processed foods and drinks (including cows', soy or other animal or dairy free milk alternatives) that are promoted to the general population, and that may be consumed by infants and young children, do not fall within the scope of this Guidance.
There is growing concern that the promotion of breastmilk substitutes and some commercial foods for infants and young children undermines optimal infant and young-child feeding.	Complementary foods have been shown to displace the intake of breastmilk if the amounts provided represent a substantial proportion of a young child's energy requirements.

What is the objective of WHO's new interpretation of 'breastmilk substitutes'?

The stated evidence for supporting the *Guidance on Ending the Inappropriate Promotion of Foods for Infants and Young Children* includes the further protection of breastfeeding, the prevention of obesity and chronic disease, and the promotion of a healthy diet.[3]

It is also stated that the guidance should encourage WHO member states to develop stronger national policies to protect children under the age of thirty-six months from marketing practices that might be detrimental to their health. It then argued that, since the adoption of the Code, manufacturers of breastmilk substitute have created 'new categories of breastmilk substitutes' in addition to traditional 'infant formulas', including 'follow-on formulas' and 'growing-up milks'. The packaging and labelling look like infant formula and are cross-promoted as such.

For their new definition of breastmilk substitutes to be logical, they need to formally recommend that mothers breastfeed for three years. Moreover, the WHO may not realize that increasing the breastfeeding period provides opportunities for industry to increase its range of milk products to cover the first three years of life – designer formulas for year one, year two, and year three – at a time when it is more important to establish infants and young children on a diverse range of complementary foods and transition to a healthy family diet.

From the perspective of families and healthcare professionals, it is important that the fundamentals of infant feeding are *unambiguous* and *evidence based*. The food sources during the early years of life are breastmilk, breastmilk substitutes and complementary foods, which are clearly defined in the Code. As recommended by WHO and UNICEF, exclusive breastfeeding should be encouraged during the first six months of life, with continued breastfeeding until two years of age or beyond, and this should be complemented by increasing quantities of safe and nutritionally adequate foods and fluids from the age of six months.[9] Preventing the inappropriate promotion of foods for infants and young children should be addressed through the provision of evidence-based composition and labelling standards. And it should be monitored by a robust regulatory process using modern technology.

From a nutrition perspective, breastmilk and breastmilk substitutes are designed to meet the total nutritional requirements of infants during the first six months of life, before introducing complementary foods. The energy and nutrient composition of the complementary foods should reflect the increasing energy and nutrient requirements of the complementary feeding period. It must be appreciated that the roles of breastmilk, infant formula and complementary foods are *different* but are also *complementary*, as clearly stated in the Code.

The impact on parents

A key argument of WHO is that inappropriate promotion of commercial complementary foods and beverages can mislead and confuse caregivers about their nutrition and health-related qualities, and about their age-appropriate and safe use. WHO also infer that such inappropriate promotion can be used to convince caregivers that family foods are inadequate, thus creating a dependence on expensive commercial products; and there is also a belief that mothers and other caregivers often do not understand the distinctions between the milk products promoted for children of different ages.[8] Parents will probably say that they fully understand what breastmilk, infant formula and solid foods are, and that they would prefer not to be confused by WHO and other organizations who appear to be creating their own language regarding infant feeding. Consider the scenario in Box 7.2.

Box 7.2: Confusion over breastmilk substitutes – breakfast options for a two-year-old child

Option 1: The mother offers a breakfast cereal that is marketed for children under three and adds a milk product that is marketed for children under three. Both products give nutritional data relating to child portion size.

Option 2: The mother offers a breakfast cereal that is not marketed for children under three and adds a milk product that is marketed for children under three. The milk gives nutritional data relating to child portion size.

Option 3: The mother offers a breakfast cereal that is marketed for children under three and adds fresh cow's milk or yogurt that is not marketed for children under three. The cereal product gives nutritional data relating to child portion size.

Option 4: The mother offers a breakfast cereal that is not marketed for children under three years and adds fresh cow's milk or yogurt that is not marketed for children under three. Neither product gives nutritional data relating to child portion size.

Now ask yourself these questions:

- For each breakfast, which foods are a breastmilk substitute or a complementary food (or both) and which are neither?
- Which option will most inform parents of the nutritional value of the breakfast?
- Which option is preferable from a public health perspective?
- How would you rate this controversy in the context of global child-health issues?

Parental opinion is highly relevant to discussions about changes in the interpretation of 'breastmilk substitutes'. If they were adequately consulted, they would undoubtedly provide a parental reality check and possible questions from parents might be along the following lines:

- Did WHO consider the distress, guilt and anger that parents may experience as a consequence of the WHO decision to describe all milk products marketed for children up to the age of three years as breastmilk substitutes?
- Is it not more logical to describe milk products that are introduced *during* the complementary feeding period as complementary foods or beverages, and milk products introduced *before* the complementary period as breastmilk substitutes?
- If milk products replace breastmilk, do other drinks and solid foods also replace breastmilk? And if they do, would this not indicate that all beverages and foods taken during the first three years should be classified as breastmilk substitutes?
- During the complementary feeding period, is the most common sequence of events that a mother decides to reduce and then stop breastfeeding, whereby the alternative product compensates for the reduction of breastmilk, and therefore does not displace breastmilk?
- Why are products that are not specifically promoted as suitable for children up to the age of three – but are commonly consumed (such as breakfast cereals that are usually accompanied by cow's milk) – not called breastmilk substitutes?
- Should products that are not promoted as being suitable for children up to the age of three years, provide a health warning for parents to this effect?

- If a mother is breastfeeding and commences her child on a milk product during the second or third year of life, is this a matter for global policy and international legislation, or should it be considered a personal decision that mothers are entitled to make with the support of a health professional?

- If WHO is concerned that labelling, branding and the use of mascots can be used to create cross-promotion of milk products – and mislead parents – will the risk of cross-promotion not be greater if all the milk products from birth to three years are classified and labelled as breastmilk substitutes?

- Would a clear separation between infant formula and complementary-feeding milk products (such as follow-up and growing-up formulas) enable a clearer understanding of their respective roles? And would this be aided by restoring the original definition of breastmilk substitutes as set out in the Code?

- Is it appropriate to make a significant change in the definition of the term breastmilk substitute without undertaking a wider review of the Code?

Preventing the inappropriate promotion of foods for infants and young children is important, but a strong lesson (learned from decades of hostility) is that actions that address the behaviour of industry should not cause collateral damage by negatively impacting on parents. In 2018, the WHO document called *Guidance on Ending the Inappropriate Promotion of Foods for Infants and Young Children. Implementation Manual,*[8] the foreword is anonymous, and there is no indication of the status of the document in terms of internal or external review, nor whether legal opinion was obtained. Its forty pages sets out the 'battle lines' that it wishes to adopt against the infant-formula industry. In effect, it calls for reinforcements from governments, particularly their legislative and enforcement functions. The content has significant implications for all stakeholders, particularly the section on law and regulation, which was driven by WHO's new understanding of what defines a breastmilk substitute. Although the document is reported to be guidance, there are requests for countries to:

- amend their existing relevant laws and/or regulations
- formulate new laws and/or regulations
- manage the legislative process
- establish processes and mechanisms for monitoring and enforcement
- develop remedial processes to correct violations

- and notably, impose sanctions that may involve the same procedures used in criminal or civil cases before the country's courts.

Referring to the battle-lines analogy, the 'generals' have to ensure they have the continued support of their 'soldiers' and the people that they serve. If such support starts to evaporate, the cause is lost. The cause to reduce the inappropriate promotion of breastmilk substitutes has been significantly harmed by the unnecessary redefining of the term breastmilk substitute. As a consequence, the troops on the ground are restless and the people they are serving are confused.

Conclusion

WHO formulated a new interpretation of the term breastmilk substitutes that is significantly different from the definition given in the Code. In its current form this interpretation lacks clarity, with blurring of the boundaries between breastmilk substitutes and complementary foods during the first three years of life. This situation creates unnecessary confusion for stakeholders, especially for families and healthcare professionals. The clear and logical definitions given in the Code should be maintained, and inappropriate promotion of the foods should be addressed through effective regulation of product composition and labelling standards. This issue has been considered in great detail in this critique, not only because it impacts on all children and their families throughout the world, but also because it raises issues of transparency, due diligence, trust and respect.

Addendum I

This chapter is based on a previously published article: Forsyth S (2018) Is WHO creating unnecessary confusion over breastmilk substitutes? *Journal of Pediatric Gastroenterology and Nutrition* 67, 760–62) The Editor of the journal invited a commentary on the article from WHO, which stimulated an exchange of correspondence that was also published in the journal, starting with: Grummer-Strawn LM (2018) Invited commentary. *Journal of Pediatric Gastroenterology and Nutrition* r6, 683. DOI: 10.1097/MPG.0000000000002137.

The exchange provides further insight to the different points of view on this important issue; the contributions are summarized in Box 7.3 over the following pages.

Box 7.3: Invited commentary and subsequent correspondence in the *Journal of Pediatric Gastroenterology and Nutrition* (2018)

Summary of the invited commentary by Grummer-Strawn (2018, r6, 683)

In the commentary, the WHO's view was that the 2016 WHO *Guidance on Ending Inappropriate Promotion of Foods for Infants and Young Children* 'clarified' the original definition contained in the Code to address ambiguities in its interpretation and they stated that: "the clarification is completely consistent with the original definition". It was also noted in the Commentary that the International Code clearly recognized that the category breast-milk substitutes is broader than just infant formula and interestingly added that:

> "... the Code provided no upper age limit on the definition of breast-milk substitutes [and] given that WHO has long recommended the continuation of breastfeeding for 2 years and beyond, it is logical that the protection of breastfeeding from inappropriate promotion of breast-milk substitutes must extend into the third year of life".

The Commentary stated that there is:

> "... a clear distinction between foods that 'replace' breastmilk (and are thereby breastmilk substitutes) and those that 'complement' breastmilk when it becomes insufficient to meet nutritional requirements. Thus distinguishing between a breastmilk substitute and a complementary food, hinges on whether the food directly reduces breastmilk consumption or adds to it".

It also stated that:

> "... the Scientific and Technical Advisory Group (STAG) that developed the recommendations concluded that there was sufficient evidence that milks targeted specifically to children under age three years do replace the intake of breast milk. Breastfeeding mothers either reduce the number of breastmilk feedings a day or stop breastfeeding altogether when other milks are introduced".

It was also noted in the Commentary that I provided no evidence to the contrary, and this is correct because there is no research evidence to determine the clinical validity of this hypothesis.

In response to my assertion that the clarification of the definition of breast-milk substitutes emerged without evidence of consultation with key stakeholders, the Commentary stated that opportunities for input across multiple stakeholders were extensive. It was argued that the draft WHO recommendations were released publicly in July 2015 along with the report from the STAG. The Commentary added that the STAG recommendations similarly stated that the scope of the Code:

"... should include any milk products (liquid or powdered) marketed for young children up to two years or beyond including follow-up formula and growing-up milks)".

The draft recommendations were made available for public comments between the last week of July and the first two weeks of August 2015, and over 300 comments were received from industry, NGOs and academics.

They added that WHO held a consultation with its member states and UN organizations in August 2015, in addition to dialogue meetings with non-governmental organizations and representatives of manufacturers of infant formula. The WHO Executive Board discussed a revised version in January 2016 and additional comments from WHO member states were reviewed in the spring of 2016. WHO concluded that throughout this process, the issue of the definition of 'breastmilk substitutes' was discussed at length and the consultation process was open and widespread.

Response to Grummer-Strawn's invited commentary (2019, 68, e41)

In my reply, the following points were noted:

"The response from Grummer-Strawn creates more questions than answers. First, he introduces some confusion on what the WHO global strategy for continued breastfeeding actually states, which is ' ... infants should receive nutritionally adequate and safe complementary foods while breastfeeding continues for up to two years of age or beyond and not 'and beyond' as he stated, and therefore for parents who have complied with the two-year breastfeeding recommendation, it will be iniquitous and illogical to designate milk products during the third year of life as breastmilk substitutes.

"Second, the STAG report did not provide an explicit recommendation on milk products being designated as breast milk substitutes up to the age of 3 years. Third, the discussion paper for the consultation process on clarification and guidance on appropriate promotion of foods did not include a recommendation that milk products up to age of 3 years should be considered as breastmilk substitutes and this issue was therefore not an integral part of the public consultation. Fourth, the WHA resolution (WHA 69.9) also made no reference to the issue of the term breastmilk substitutes being extended to the age of 3 years. Fifth, to meet the increasing energy and nutrient requirements in early life there

needs to be a transition from breast milk to more nutrient dense complementary foods, and this inevitably involves complementary foods replacing breast milk, as the WHO has previously detailed. As Grummer-Strawn declares that he alone is responsible for the views expressed in his response an official communication from the WHO on this matter would be most welcome."

Response from Grummer-Strawn (2019, 68, e41–42)

"In my Commentary, I did not provide a specific quote from any single document, but Forsyth is correct that the Global Strategy for Infant and Young Child Feeding does use the wording '2 years of age or beyond' not 'and beyond'. This distinction may be important for an individual mother deciding whether she has continued breastfeeding 'long enough'. But the protection of breastfeeding must be in place both before and after 2 years of age if mothers are to decide on the 'or beyond' without commercial pressure.

"Although the STAG report did not spell out the cut-off of 3 years, it clearly stated that follow-up formula and growing-up milks should be included in the scope of the code. The Codex Alimentarius Standard for Follow up Formula (CXS 156- 1987) defines follow-up formula as a liquid food for infants from the sixth month on and for young children, and it defines young children as 'persons from the age of more than 12 months up to the age of 3 years (36 months)'. The WHO consultation Discussion Paper similarly said that growing-up milks should be considered breastmilk substitutes and cited Codex for definitions. In response to requests from Member States and other reviewers, the final version of the Guidance made the language clearer without altering the meaning.

"World Health Assembly resolutions do not typically restate the recommendations in the documents they cite or comment on. In this case, there was no reason to do so, because the assembly called on governments to implement the recommendations contained in the guidance.

"To meet their increasing energy and nutrient requirements in early life, young children need to consume nutrient-dense complementary foods in addition to breastmilk. The Guiding Principles on Complementary Feeding of the Breastfed Child clearly indicate that breastfeeding makes an important nutritional contribution after 6 months of age but that 'other foods and liquids are needed, along with breast milk'. In no place does the document suggest that other milks should replace breast milk. WHO's position on this issue was clearly stated in the 2016 guidance. Subsequently, additional documents have been posted on the WHO website to provide further clarity and rationale."

For health policy-making processes to be credible there needs to be due diligence, inclusivity and clinical relevance. From the above correspondence, I would like to point out the following.

First, a lack of due diligence. The three-year rule attached to the change in the definition of breastmilk substitutes was achieved without being specifically mentioned in the STAG report, the consultation document, or WHA resolution 69.9. This is surprising because the term 'breastmilk substitute' is a key element of all infant-feeding policies and is the source of much debate between stakeholders.

Second, the photograph of WHO officials, members of IBFAN and the Chair of the Working Group (Fig. 7.1) celebrating the outcome of WHA resolution 69.9 (http://www.babymilkaction.org/archives/9771) gives the impression of *collusion* rather than *collaboration* or simply *consultation*, with other stakeholders such as scientists, clinicians, and parents being excluded. WHO should be seen to be representing the views and interests of all stakeholders.

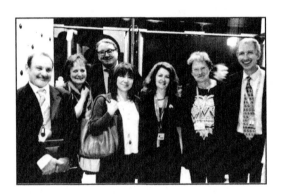

Fig. 7.1: Photograph showing representatives from WHO and IBFAN and the Chair of the WHO Working Group celebrating the passage of the WHO Resolution (WHA 69.9) at the World Health Assembly in 2016, in which the WHO guidance document included the redefinition of the term 'breastmilk substitute'.

Third, extending the term 'breastmilk substitute' to children up to the age of three is more likely to increase the sales of formula milk as companies increase their range of 'designer' formulas for this extended period. Rather than concentrating on a liquid diet during this period, the focus should be on extending the range of nutritious complementary foods. In the above correspondence the WHO commented that no age limit was applied to breastmilk substitutes within the Code.

Finally, I have to ask, why is this topic a policy-making priority for WHO when there are significantly greater concerns such as severe malnutrition, stunting and the double burden of malnutrition? What are the anticipated health benefits of the new definition of 'breastmilk substitute' if it is likely to be associated with increased sales of formula milk, and have a negative impact on transitioning to a healthy family diet – and be greeted by parents with disbelief?

Addendum II

The Codex Alimentarius CCNFSDU met in November 2019 to finalize the composition standards for follow-up formula. There were long discussions on the nomenclature for these formulas and similar products. Interestingly, it was concluded that decisions about what is considered a breastmilk substitute should be decided at a country level, rather than the Codex document stating whether or not a product should be labelled as a breastmilk substitute. As part of the effort to reduce the confusion of consumers, it was suggested that the words 'formula', 'growing-up milk' and 'formulated' should not be used. The Codex document now recommends that milk products for children aged twelve months to three years should have a 'neutral' name – either a 'drink for young children' or a 'drink with added nutrients'. This allows individual countries to choose which term to use in their national legislation.

WHO primarily focuses on protecting, promoting and supporting breastfeeding, whereas the primary objective of the Codex Alimentarius is the protection of *consumers*. Attendees at their meetings are not limited to government representatives. They include a broader range of observers, including academics, health professionals, NGOs and industry representatives. WHO is also represented at these meetings but clearly the outcome of the discussion did not reflect their views, and therefore their proposed 'clarification' of the term 'breastmilk substitute' appears to lack general support.

There is another complication of this self-inflicted intervention by WHO. In order to progress legislation pertaining to breastmilk substitutes, it will be necessary to have an agreed legally binding definition of the term 'breastmilk substitutes'. WHO's intervention on redefining a breastmilk substitute has now seriously jeopardized the possibility of a global consensus being achieved.

References

1.   WHO (1981) *International Code of Marketing of Breastmilk Substitutes.* Available at: https://apps.who.int/iris/bitstream/handle/10665/40382/9241541601. pdf?sequence=1&isAllowed=y (last accessed August 2022).

2.   WHO (2016) Maternal, infant, and young child nutrition. *Guidance on Ending the Inappropriate Promotion of Foods for Infants and Young Children. 69th WHA*

Document A69/7 Add.1 2016. Available at: http://apps.who.int/gb/ebwha/pdf_files/ WHA69/A69_7Add1-en.pdf?ua=1&ua=1/ (last accessed August 2022).

3. _WHO (2015) *Draft clarification and guidance on inappropriate promotion of foods for infants and young children: Report of the Scientific and Technical Advisory Group (STAG) on inappropriate promotion of foods for infants and young children.* Available at: https://cdn.who.int/media/docs/default-source/nutritionlibrary/complementary-feeding/stag-report-inappropriate-promotion-infant-foods-en.pdf?sfvrsn=69120e6a_2 (last accessed August 2022).

4. WHA (2016) *Ending inappropriate promotion of foods for infants and young children. WHA 69.9.* Available at: http://apps.who.int/gb/ebwha/pdf_files/WHA69/A69_R9–en.pdf (last accessed August 2022).

5. WHO/UNICEF (2018) *Information note: clarification on the classification of follow-up formulas for children 6–36 months as breast milk substitutes.* Available at: https://www.who.int/publications/i/item/WHO-NMH-NHD-18.11 (last accessed August 2022).

6. Codex Alimentarius (2017) *Guidelines on formulated complementary foods for older infants and young children. CAC/GL 8–1991.* Adopted in 1991. Amended in 2017. Revised in 2013. Available at: https://www.fao.org/fao–who–codexalimentarius/sh–proxy/zh/?lnk=1&url=https%253A%252F%252Fworkspace.fao.org%252Fsites%252Fcodex%252FStandards%252FCXG%2B8–1991%252FCXG_008e.pdf (last accessed August 2022).

7. WHO (2001) *Report of the Expert Consultation on the optimal duration of exclusive breastfeeding.* Available at: https://apps.who.int/iris/bitstream/handle/10665/67219/WHO_NHD_01.09.pdf?ua=1 (last accessed August (2022).

8. WHO (2017) *Guidance on ending the inappropriate promotion of foods for infants and young children. Implementation Manual.* Licence: CC BY-NC-SA 3.0 IGO. Available at: https://apps.who.int/iris/bitstream/handle/10665/260137/978924 1513470-eng.pdf (last accessed August 2022).

9. WHO/UNICEF (2003) *Global strategy for infant and young-child feeding.* Available at: http://apps.who.int/iris/bitstream/10665/42590/1/9241562218.pdf?ua=1&ua=1 (last accessed August 2022).

CHAPTER 8

How critical is the duration of continued breastfeeding for child health?

Relating the health benefits of breastfeeding to the duration of breastfeeding is important from a policy perspective as it can provide parents with evidence upon which they can decide how long they wish to breastfeed their children. However, providing specific and relevant information can be problematic. To be of value to specific families, the data need to be derived from an appropriate population, reflecting socioeconomic, demographic and geographic characteristics. The quality of research must be carefully considered because randomized controlled trials (RCTs) of breastfeeding are unethical, and observational studies can be complicated by known and unknown confounding variable factors. In the absence of the most robust evidence, decision-making may be subject to opinion rather than evidence or fact.

Evidence or opinion?

It is not always clear whether a particular health outcome is directly related to breastfeeding or whether it is an indirect association. A statistical association between two variables merely implies that knowing the value of one variable provides information about the value of the other. It does not necessarily mean that one *causes* the other.

It is possible that there may be a single association for a single condition, but in practice this would be unusual, and even in that situation causation may not be confirmed. More commonly there are several factors that are associated with a particular condition, many of which may be associated with other conditions, and these conditions may have an association with the primary condition that is being considered. With breastfeeding, it is important to reflect on the many conditions relating to a mother or her infant that have been associated with breastfeeding and determine whether there is clear direct evidence of causation. Association should *never* be confused with causation. For example, an association between the duration of breastfeeding with childhood obesity or maternal breast cancer should not be immediately interpreted to mean that breastfeeding prevents these conditions. This issue is discussed further in Chapters 9 and 11. Taking the relationship between breastfeeding, childhood obesity and maternal breast cancer as examples, it is evident that classifying a relationship as an association or a causation can be complex. This is illustrated in Box 8.1.

Box 8.1: Potential interconnections between maternal breastfeeding and (a) childhood obesity and (b) maternal breast cancer

(a) Childhood obesity

- Breastfeeding is associated with a decreased risk of childhood obesity.
- Maternal obesity is associated with childhood obesity.
- Maternal weight gain during pregnancy is associated with childhood obesity.
- Maternal preconception obesity is associated with childhood obesity.
- Maternal obesity is associated with a decreased prevalence of breastfeeding.

(b) Maternal breast cancer

- Maternal breastfeeding is associated with a decreased risk of maternal breast cancer.
- Maternal obesity is associated with an increased risk of breast cancer.
- Maternal obesity is associated with a decreased prevalence of breastfeeding.
- There are health, socioeconomic, and lifestyle factors associated with breast cancer.
- There are health, socioeconomic, and lifestyle factors associated with obesity.
- There are health, socioeconomic, and lifestyle factors associated with breastfeeding.
- The same factors may be associated with breastfeeding, obesity, and breast cancer.
- Causation needs scientific evidence of plausible mechanisms.
- Plausible mechanisms of causation need to be confirmed by direct experimental studies.

To clarify the scientific validity of an association, the possible underlying mechanisms must be identified, and then individually tested in well-conducted experimental studies. Moreover, before obtaining greater clarity on the relationship of breastfeeding to breast cancer, or any other condition, it is important for policymakers, breastfeeding activist groups, health professionals and parents to understand the limitations of the breastfeeding data that is available, and judgements have to be carefully balanced with the *level* of evidence available. From the perspective of parents, unsubstantiated information may be distressing and harmful. This is discussed in more detail in Chapter 11.

It is recognized that separating evidence from opinion can often be difficult, but at all times the recipients (e.g. parents) should be assured that any exchange of information meets acceptable standards of honesty and transparency. In an attempt to bring clarification on 'evidence' and 'opinion', a recent article in the *British Medical Journal* defined them thus:[1]

- *Evidence*—facts intended for use in support of a conclusion
- *Opinion*—a view or judgement formed about something, not necessarily based on facts.

From these definitions it is clear that determining what is evidence and what is opinion may not be straightforward – discussions on the subject may generate many opinions but offer few facts, and therefore not be considered as evidence.

There is a common view that medicine is not an exact science, and some consider it an art, the underlying assertion being that the best clinicians are not only skilled and knowledgeable but also have astute clinical judgement.[2] This is relevant in policymaking as the highest quality of evidence may not be available to underpin policies, and in these circumstances the discussion centres on whether the available evidence is 'good enough' for a policy or guideline – and that is a matter of judgement. So, for policies on infant feeding (whether global, national or community-based) it is important to determine whether the evidence is 'good enough' or whether the policy is light on evidence and heavy on opinion.

Establishing evidence on breastfeeding and child health

The validity of a health policy may stand or fall on the strength of the evidence of health benefit. The list of health benefits reported to relate to breastfeeding continues to grow; positive effects are reported from infancy through to late adult life. In 2007, the US Agency for Healthcare Research and Quality (AHRQ) published a summary of systematic reviews and meta-analyses on breastfeeding and maternal and infant health outcomes in developed countries.[3] There are reports of an association between infant breastfeeding and several conditions throughout the lifespan, such as:

- in early life, with a reduction in gastrointestinal, respiratory and ear infections, and a lower risk of sudden infant death syndrome (SIDS)
- in later childhood, with a reduction in lower respiratory tract infections, asthma and leukaemia
- in adulthood, with a reduction in type 2 diabetes, cardiovascular disease and mental health disorders.

And mothers who breastfeed are reported to have reduced risks of hormone-related cancers, including breast and ovarian.

However, the AHRQ cautioned that, although a history of breastfeeding is associated with a reduced risk of many diseases in infants and mothers, almost all the data in their review were gathered from observational studies and there was wide variation in its quality. Thus, the associations described in the report do not necessarily represent *causality*. Any associations between breastfeeding and health outcomes are complex and overinterpretation should be avoided.

It is well documented that the demographic, socioeconomic, health and education characteristics of women who choose to breastfeed are quite different from those who choose to formula-feed. Similarly, there are differences between women who start breastfeeding then stop after a short period and those who breastfeed for longer. Recent data suggest that the *pre*-pregnant health status of a mother is the causal link to their future health, and the decision to breastfeed is a marker of better pre-pregnant health.[4] Thus the positive health effects may be overestimated if pre-pregnant health status is not considered in studies of the long-term health effects of breastfeeding.

In relation to the association of child intelligence with breastfeeding, a large US population study reported that maternal IQ was more highly predictive of breastfeeding status than race, education, age, poverty status, smoking, home environment, or a child's birth weight or birth order.[5] One standard-deviation advantage in maternal IQ more than doubled the odds of the mother choosing to breastfeed. Before adjustment, breastfeeding was associated with an increase of around four points in child cognitive ability. Adjustment for maternal IQ accounted for most of this effect and, when fully adjusted for a range of relevant confounders, the effect was small (0.52 points) and statistically insignificant.[5]

A separate analysis of a subgroup of siblings living in the same environment also showed no significant difference in cognitive ability between breastfed and formula-fed children.[5] The authors concluded that:

> *"…breastfeeding has little or no effect on intelligence in children. While breastfeeding has many advantages for the child and mother, enhancement of intelligence is unlikely to be among them".*

If an infant and young-child feeding policy is to cover the period from birth to the age of three years, reliable data is required about the continuum of diet during the three-year period that can be related to the health outcomes being studied. For example, does exclusive breastfeeding, or continued breastfeeding for two years or beyond, or introducing complementary foods at around six months, or progressing to a nutritious family diet, individually or collectively influence the risk of obesity, high blood pressure or cognitive function in later life? The answer is that we do not know.

The focus of most studies has been on breastfeeding, but many of them compare different durations of exclusive, predominant and partial breastfeeding and different complementary feeding practices (if included), and different durations of continuous breastfeeding (if included). There are usually no data on establishing a family diet. Many of these studies are observational, in which there may be a high degree of statistical wizardry, with re-profiling of incomplete data and adjustments made for a multitude of known and potentially unknown confounding factors. In studies that limit their investigation to the first year of life and relate breastfeeding to early-life health outcomes (such as gastrointestinal and respiratory illnesses) the recall of information is more accurate for feeding data and history of illness – but when relating later health to infant feeding history the reliability of data may be suspect.

In 2013, WHO commissioned a review of the long-term health effects of breastfeeding, a follow-up to a previous review from 2007. It was undertaken by Horta and Victora, who focused on overweightness and obesity, blood pressure, cholesterol, cognitive function, diabetes type 2 and blood pressure.[6] The authors commented:

> *"The meta-analyses of overweight/obesity, blood pressure, diabetes and intelligence suggest that benefits are larger for children and adolescents, and smallest among adults, suggesting a gradual dilution of the effect with time. Because the meta-analyses are almost exclusively based on observational studies the possibility of self-selection and residual confounding must be considered. Even when multiple studies show similar results, these studies may largely be subject to the same biases. In particular, most studies are derived from high-income settings where*

breastfeeding is more common among highly educated, more affluent mothers who are more health conscious, and whose offspring may be less likely to suffer from the negative outcomes covered in the present review. The fact that estimates from high-quality studies, with tighter control of confounding, are less marked than those from all studies suggests that this may be the case".

The authors referred to the only two randomized studies on the subject – one a follow-up study of preterm infants in England allocated to breast or formula milk in early life,[7,8] and the Belarus PROBIT trial, in which mothers were allocated to a breastfeeding-promotion intervention (discussed in detail below).[9-15] They interpreted the results of their meta-analyses of 2007 and 2013 and the two randomized trials as shown in Table 8.1.

It is important to note Horta and Victora's cautious interpretation of the data. They acknowledged the weakness of observational data and the influence of unknown confounders, as well as some basic methodological differences, for example, in the criteria used for the breastfeeding groups. This level of caution contrasts with the more assertive, definitive approach of WHO and breastfeeding interest groups, who often translate weak associations between breastfeeding and clinical conditions as 'cause and effect', and claim that breastfeeding is 'protective', or 'prevents' or 'reduces'. There is a fine balance between providing information that is important for parents and providing information that is *not* 'good enough'.

Footnote to Table 8.1 (opposite)

*More recent data from the PROBIT study show that children aged 6.5, 11.5 and 16 years who are exclusively breastfed for six months versus three months, had statistically significantly higher mean values for BMI, triceps skinfold thickness and hip circumference, but no significant differences in height.7

**An intention-to-treat (ITT) analysis in the PROBIT study shows that at 6.5 years the cluster-adjusted difference in verbal IQ was significantly higher by 7.5 points in the breastfeeding-promotion intervention group, and the verbal subtests were also significantly higher than in the control group. There were no significant differences in non-verbal subtests, performance IQ or the cluster-adjusted difference in full-scale IQ. At 16 years, the advantage in verbal IQ was reduced to 1.4 points and no differences were noted in the ITT analysis for the exclusive breastfeeding for three- or six-months' groups.8 It is therefore commented that the early effects did not continue into adolescence.

Table 8.1: Summary of results from two meta-analyses by Horta and Victora (2007 and 2013).

Outcome	Summary of finding
Total cholesterol	The 2007 meta-analysis found a significant effect on cholesterol levels among adults, but the 2013 did not. The UK randomized trial of preterm infants showed a small protective effect, but the Belarus trial did not. *Conclusion:* Breastfeeding does not appear to reduce total cholesterol levels.
Blood pressure	The pooled meta-analyses indicated a small reduction (less than 1 mmHg) in systolic pressure among breastfed infants, but no significant change in diastolic pressure. Other confounding factors may be important here. The two randomized trials found no association with breastfeeding. *Conclusion:* Any protective effect of breastfeeding may be too small to be of significance.
Diabetes type 2	The pooled meta-analyses showed a substantial (34%) reduction in the incidence of type-2 diabetes, but only a few studies were available and their results were highly variable. Only two high-quality studies were identified and these had conflicting results – one found an increase in incidence of diabetes and the other a decrease. Neither of the two randomized trials gave results for this outcome. *Conclusion:* Further studies are needed in this area.
Over-weight/ obesity	The pooled meta-analyses showed that breastfeeding was associated with a 24% reduction in overweight/obesity. The two high-quality trials showed only a 12% reduction. Confounding factors may still be at play because no protection was evident in studies from low- and middle-income countries, where the social patterning of breastfeeding is not clearcut. The PROBIT trial did not find an association. *Conclusion:* Breastfeeding may provide some protection against overweight/obesity, but confounding factors cannot be ruled out.*
Intelligence tests	The pooled meta-analyses found that breastfeeding was associated with an increase of 3.5 points in normalized test scores, and 2.2 points if only the high-quality studies were included. The two randomized trials found significant effects, providing strong albeit modest) evidence of a causal effect of breastfeeding on IQ.** *Conclusion:* Later data from PROBIT cast doubt on longer term benefit.

More on the Belarus PROBIT study

PROBIT has been described as the largest randomized controlled study of human lactation. The primary objective was to determine whether a breastfeeding-support initiative prolonged breastfeeding duration. The secondary aim was to investigate whether longer duration and exclusivity was associated with improved health outcomes from birth to adolescence. The study was unique because of its randomized design for intervention and control arms, and because it gathered prospective data over sixteen years from a large sample of participants, with a relatively low attrition (drop out) rate.[9-15] It generated a series of publications, the most recent of which providing health outcome data on participants at the age of 16 years. A key element of the trial was the repetition of assessments at different time periods, which has provided some clarity on whether the early identifiable effects of prolonged breastfeeding are persistent or transient.

Note that it is considered unethical to randomize individual women in breastfeeding-intervention studies, hence the researchers took the novel approach of establishing a randomized controlled trial to compare the impact of a promotion intervention on pregnant women with a comparable group receiving standard care.

Design and methodology

This large cluster-randomized trial was led by researchers from Canada, the UK and USA, but conducted in the (former Soviet) Republic of Belarus, where hospital and outpatient settings were considered not to be 'breastfeeding friendly', and thus responsive to the intervention. The intervention was based on the Baby-Friendly Hospital Initiative (BFHI) that was developed by WHO and UNICEF to promote and support breastfeeding particularly among mothers who choose to initiate breastfeeding. A total of 17,046 mother–infant pairs were enrolled at thirty-one cluster sites. Of these, only 555 (3.3%) were lost to follow-up during the first year. To reduce potential bias from low adherence to the randomization, all outcomes were analyzed on an intention-to-treat (ITT) principle – that is, by comparison of the two randomized groups (intervention and control). There were also observational studies, undertaken specifically to investigate the effects of exclusive breastfeeding for 3 months or less, 3-6 months and 6 months or more. Of the entire cohort, 2862 infants were exclusively breastfed for three months, and 621 were exclusively breastfed for six months or more. When the study was designed, the official WHO recommendation for exclusive breastfeeding was four to six months.

Breastfeeding duration

The initial component of the trial met the primary objective by demonstrating that a breastfeeding-promotion initiative successfully extends the period of breastfeeding: 19.7% of mothers in the intervention group continued to breast feed at twelve months compared to 11.4% in the control group and were more likely to exclusively breastfeed at three months (43.3% vs 6.4%) and at six months (7.9% versus 0.6%).[11]

Gastrointestinal infections

During the first year of life, the ITT analysis showed that fewer infants in the intervention group experienced more than one gastrointestinal infection versus controls (9.1% and 13.2%, respectively),[11] and showed a 40% reduction in infections in the intervention group. The pattern was similar in the observational data, whereby gastrointestinal infection was reported in 7.4% of infants receiving three months exclusive breastfeeding compared to 5.0% of infants exclusively fed for six months. However, both types of analyses showed no significant differences in hospital admissions due to gastrointestinal infection, suggesting that the duration and exclusivity of breastfeeding did not reduce the risk of severity. For time periods of birth to three months, three to six months and more than six months, the beneficial effect was only evident in the three- to six-month group.

Note that the researchers use the term 'gastrointestinal infection' but like similar studies they did not provide microbiological data to confirm the presence of infection. Diagnosis was based on the presence of at least two of the following symptoms: increased stool frequency, loose stools, vomiting, and temperature greater than 38.5 °C.

Other infections

During the first year of life, the ITT analysis found no significant difference between intervention and control groups for upper respiratory tract infection, otitis media, croup, wheezing or pneumonia. There were also no differences found between the groups fed exclusively for three months and six months.[11]

Neurocognitive function

Cognitive function assessed at 6.5 years using the seven components of the Wechsler Abbreviated Scales of Intelligence. In the ITT analysis, the cluster-adjusted difference in verbal IQ was significantly higher (7.5 points) in the intervention group. The verbal subtests were also significantly higher. However, there was no significant difference in the non-verbal subtests, and no difference between the groups for performance IQ or the cluster-adjusted difference in full-scale IQ.[10] Comparisons were also made of the exclusively breast fed for three-months and six-months groups. The seven Wechsler assessments and another five assessments (teachers' ratings) found no difference between the two groups.

At 16 years of age, the advantage in verbal function reduced to 1.4 points (from 7.9 points at age 6.5), but no difference was noted in the non-verbal subtests or between the groups for full-scale IQ.[10] The mechanisms underlying this diluted effect of breastfeeding on cognition at a later age are unclear, but the authors speculated that other environmental factors (such as school characteristics, peer influence and parental intellectual stimulation) become more important as children grow older. They also noted that studies of infant feeding (breastmilk versus pre-term formula and pre-term versus standard formula) report that early diet is more strongly associated with language development. Nutrients in breastmilk, such as the long chain omega-3 and omega-6 fatty acids (docosahexaenoic acid (DHA) and arachidonic acid (ARA), respectively), may be beneficial for cognitive development, which has been found in some – but not all – studies, but the mechanisms relating DHA to verbal function have not been reported.

The PROBIT authors speculated that the better verbal function in early life among breastfed children may be due to greater maternal responsiveness, psychological bonding or frequency of verbal exchange during breastfeeding, as compared with bottle-feeding, and perhaps relates to the increased duration and frequency of feeding sessions.

Childhood weight gain

At 6.5 years, the ITT analysis showed no significant effects of the intervention leading to longer breastfeeding on height, body mass index (BMI), waist and hip circumference, or triceps and subscapular skinfold thickness.[13,14] However, children in the six-months exclusive breastfeeding group had statistically significant higher mean values for BMI, triceps skinfold thickness, and hip circumference (but no significant differences in height) than those in the three-month group.[9] At age 11.5, the ITT analysis showed increased hip circumference and BMI in the intervention group.[15] In the observational analyses, increased duration of exclusive breastfeeding was associated with increased body mass, fat mass and fat-free mass indices, hip circumference, head and mid-upper arm circumference, and overweight/obesity.[12] At age 16, similar trends were noted for weight and BMI.[14] The PROBIT authors concluded that the intervention did

118

not prevent overweight/obesity; in fact, it was slightly more prevalent in the intervention arm. While there are many reasons for promoting breastfeeding in terms of duration and exclusivity, the authors state that "*their data do not indicate that breastfeeding prevents obesity during childhood or adolescence*".

Cardiovascular and metabolic factors

At age 6.5, 11.5 and 16 years, the ITT analysis found no difference in systolic or diastolic blood pressure between the intervention and control groups.[12] The observational studies comparing three versus six months exclusive breastfeeding also showed no significant difference in blood pressure at these age points. Metabolic outcomes at 11.5 years included those related to the development of diabetes, namely glucose and insulin levels, insulin resistance, and two markers for the development of cardiovascular disease, adiponectin and ApoA1. Results from both the ITT and observational analyses indicate that the mean values of all these measures, and the prevalence of metabolic syndrome, were similar in the intervention and control groups. The researchers concluded that the significant improvements in duration and exclusivity of breastfeeding in the intervention group did not reduce measures of insulin resistance or cardiometabolic risk at 11.5 years. In fact, the estimates were generally in the opposite direction to the hypothesized protective effects, and the confidence intervals were reported to be consistent with chance or small-intervention effects. The researchers noted that the absence of a favourable effect on blood pressure at 11.5 years is similar to the results at age 6.5 years and is consistent with the lack of impact of prolonged exclusive breastfeeding on general and peripheral adiposity at age 11.5. They stated that their findings do not support previous studies which suggest that increased exclusivity and duration of breastfeeding is associated with reduced cardiometabolic risk factors.[14]

Atopic eczema and wheezing

During the first year of life, the occurrence of atopic eczema rashes was reduced by 46% in the intervention group, with a similar reduction in non-eczematous rashes.[13,15] The ITT analysis showed a substantial and significantly lower risk of atopic eczema with the intervention. The observational results suggested that exclusive breastfeeding for three months (with continued breastfeeding for six months or more) provided a similar level of protection against atopic eczema to six months' exclusive breastfeeding. At 6.5 years, no difference was found between the three-month and six-month exclusive-breastfeeding groups for eczema, wheezing, asthma and a variety of allergy tests,[13,15] and the intervention group showed no reduction in risk of allergic symptoms and diagnoses or positive skin-prick tests. Thus, the results do not support a protective effect of prolonged and exclusive breastfeeding on asthma or allergy.

PROBIT's contribution to policy-making

How do these data contribute to current and future policy-making? The strengths of this large longitudinal trial include its randomization, impressive sample size, and the good retention of participants. The extensive body of data demonstrates how outcome measures change with time, as the effects of early diet diminish and other health and lifestyle factors come into play.

The choice of location was also important. At the time of recruitment, Belarus was a medium-income country with established national health and education systems. The availability of water and food was adequate and childhood obesity and ill-health rates were low. Previous studies on the health effects of breastfeeding tended to be undertaken in countries in which utilities were seriously deficient, childhood malnutrition was severe, and breastfeeding was prolonged. There is well-documented evidence that prolonged breastfeeding saves lives in these circumstances, but it is also known that adequate complementary feeding saves more lives, and malnutrition and stunting are reduced.

Other studies have been carried out in more affluent countries, in which breastfeeding duration is relatively short. Mortality is low but obesity-related morbidity is high, but this may relate to the quantity and quality of complementary foods and family diet.

Surprisingly, WHO officials have been reluctant to refer to the PROBIT data – apart from the initial results on gastrointestinal illness in the first year of life, which was key evidence in the original consultation process for the 2003 global infant-feeding strategy document.

The PROBIT study may not be perfect in design as the randomization related to the breastfeeding promotion intervention and participants were not individually randomized to short or prolonged breastfeeding which would be unethical. However, it was a large, randomized trial that collected prospective data over a sixteen-year period on short and longer breastfeeding periods, with outcomes measured in over thirty health-related domains – clearly valuable information with relevance to policy-making. The data were generated by three highly respected international research teams, resulting in the publication of over forty scientific papers in more than twenty high-impact scientific journals, and under the scrutiny of at least twenty editorial boards and around eighty external reviewers. It therefore remains a mystery that WHO are so reluctant to highlight the information gleaned in the relevant documents.

Breastfeeding in the second year of life

Evidence about the effect of breastfeeding in the second year of life is very limited, despite WHO's global recommendation of continuing breastfeeding for two years or beyond, which was first recorded in the Innocenti Declaration in 1990. In 2018, WHO produced an Information Note to provide "*clarification on the classification of follow-up formulas for children 6–36 months as breastmilk substitutes*".[16]

The purpose of the Note was to retrospectively explain the rationale for the WHA recommendation that milk products marketed for children up to three years of age should be understood to be 'breastmilk substitutes'. The focus of the Note on child health related to the claim that breastfeeding for more than one-year reduced child mortality and protected against childhood overweightness.

The effect of breastfeeding on child mortality was based on a systematic review published in 2015,[17] which included six observational studies on breastfeeding for twelve to twenty-three months published between 1986 and 1996, originating from Guinea-Bissau, Pakistan, Philippines, Ghana, Senegal and Gambia, in which the participants predominantly lived in rural areas in overcrowded homes. The WHO Information Note stated:

> "*Continued breastfeeding in the second year of life protects against mortality, with children who are not breastfed at 12–23 months of age being twice as likely to die compared to those who are breastfed in the second year of life*".

Several factors call the validity of this statement into question. The data, published as part of the 2015 systematic review and highlighted by WHO in 2018, were from observational studies, conducted in some of the former poorest countries in the world. How relevant are these data for global policies in the 2020s and beyond? The majority of the global target population lives in significantly changed circumstances today, and it is hoped that the socioeconomic conditions of the original six populations has now improved, if they have not, then that should be the focus of the Note. It is odd that it carries WHO's logo, but the authors' names are not given, nor is there is any evidence of external review, which contrasts with the standards required by peer-reviewed scientific journals. In relation to the effect of breastfeeding duration in the second year of life on overweight/ obesity, the Note refers to a systematic review published in 2005 that included seventeen studies, all from developed countries, but only one of them included a breastfeeding category of > 12 months. This was a large population study and it did not include information on complementary feeding.[18] The Note concluded that the protection of breastfeeding against childhood overweightness is the strongest for infants who are breastfed for more than a year, however, it is reported in the publication that:

> *"From 1 month of breastfeeding onward, the risk of subsequent overweight continuously decreased up to a reduction of more than 30 percent, reaching a plateau at 9 months of breastfeeding".*

As an official communication advising on prolonged breastfeeding, the evidence is weak, and the presentation lacks the editorial standards that are expected for professional and scientific publications.

Is this information an appropriate or inappropriate promotion of breastfeeding? Is it evidence or is it opinion? Opinions should be listened to, naturally, especially at the stage of developing research ideas that may progress to formal research and ultimately provide an evidence base for national and international policy. But in some aspects of infant feeding, opinion appears to be translated into global policy with the briefest possible reference to research, or strength of evidence. A key message from the Note is the obvious lack of contemporary studies to support WHO's recommended continuing-breastfeeding policy. This may reflect a reluctance of researchers and clinicians to become involved in the field of infant-feeding research, who may instead shift their talents to research environments in which they are welcomed and supported.

Alignment of research and advocacy

Advocacy activities should be grounded in evidence. To achieve this, researchers should be actively involved in ensuring that advocacy interventions are informed and appropriate. Unjustified claims often result from genuine misunderstandings, or poor translation of knowledge, however motivational bias is also a possible factor. Researchers can support advocacy efforts by providing clear evidence summaries and speaking up when findings are inappropriately used for advocacy. In addition, they can contribute by evaluating advocacy strategies to objectively determine their efficacy.

An excellent review of perceived barriers and challenges to infant-feeding research addressed some key areas to which scientists may more effectively contribute.[19]

These include:

- the importance of collaborating across disciplines and beyond traditional partnerships
- the use of rigorous study designs to mitigate bias
- the need to capture and study modern feeding practices
- the value of evaluating human milk as a whole rather than a mixture of discrete components
- the need to develop and adapt messaging for diverse stakeholders
- the importance of challenging unsubstantiated claims by any stakeholder
- actively participating in public policy development.

It is anticipated that greater alignment between research and advocacy may not only reduce conflicting messages from key stakeholders but also ultimately enable improved working relations between them.

Conclusion

Despite inconsistencies in the data, a pragmatic view is that breastfeeding during the first year of life offers health benefits in early and later childhood. However, there is only limited evidence of its health benefits in children who were breastfed during the second year of life. There is evidence of health benefits to mothers, which will be discussed in Chapter 11.

To enable future progress and consolidate our understanding of optimal infant and young-child feeding, there needs to be more effective planning and coordination of research activities. This will ensure that lessons are learned from the many studies with deficient designs and methodologies. There are several initiatives where national and international advisory and monitoring research centres have been set up to coordinate and monitor research activities on a specific aspect of clinical research and this has led to improvement in the quality of studies and provided a strategic direction that has led to improvements in health outcomes.

It is strongly recommended, therefore, that consideration is given to a Global Research Advisory Centre for infant and child nutrition. It would play an advisory and monitoring role for all researchers planning to undertake scientific and clinical research on the health benefits of infant and young-child feeding. Its objectives would be to promote infant and young-child feeding as an important and exciting area of clinical research, and to ensure that there is learning from past experiences and thus an improvement in the quality of future projects and publications. It would also strategically prioritize the key areas of research, disseminate study results, provide accurate interpretations and fact checking of data, inform messaging by stakeholder and consumer groups, and make sure the reputations of researchers from both academia and industry are protected from inappropriate criticism.

Addendum

Professor Michael Kramer, from McGill University, Canada was the Principal Investigator for the PROBIT study, and he and his research team conducted the study in Belarus. As his research studies and his systematic reviews of the literature on the health benefits of breastfeeding, have directly contributed to the current WHO global policies on healthcare, I wished to hear from him directly about his current thinking on WHO breastfeeding policy and the best advice for parents. Our exchanges are reproduced here (Box 8.2) with his consent (where the abbreviations BF and EBF stand for breastfeeding and exclusive breastfeeding, respectively; GI is gastrointestinal, and SIDS is sudden infant death syndrome).

Box 8.2: Unpublished correspondence with Professor Michael Kramer of the PROBIT study (2014)

First letter (10 July 2014)

I continue to follow the data arising from the Belarus Study with great interest. The duration of exclusive breastfeeding is a frequent discussion point at meetings with parents, and I am often asked for evidence that exclusive breastfeeding for 6 months confers additional health gain compared to exclusive breastfeeding for 4 months. As you will be aware only 1% of mothers in the UK exclusively breastfeed for 6 months and almost certainly it is the most non-compliant of all public health policies. The view of parents is that they fully understand the potential benefits of exclusive breastfeeding for 6 months or longer in countries where sanitation is poor, the water supply is contaminated and literacy rates are low, but they do not understand why the same policy should apply when the population is literate, they live in an environment with good sanitation and houses are supplied with a clean water. Clearly it is imperative that health policies engender a sense of ownership within the target population and for this to be achieved the evidence needs to be honest, transparent and robust. For that reason, I would welcome your response to a question that is increasingly being raised: In a medium to high economy society where literacy rates are high, sanitation is good and the water supply is clean, is there evidence that 6 months exclusive breastfeeding provides unequivocal additional health gain to the infant compared to the infant who receives exclusive breastfeeding for 4 months.

I appreciate that any discussion about duration of exclusive breastfeeding is potentially sensitive, but I also believe that we need to ensure that the message to parents is explicit and based on fact. Moreover, it is important to ensure that public health policies meet scientific, professional and ethical standards. I would be extremely grateful if you could find time to respond and I look forward to your thoughts on this important public health issue.

Response from Professor Kramer (14 July 2014)

I understand your question, and it's one I've heard repeatedly from journalists (especially those from the UK!), other scientists, and even mothers. I've attached our two PROBIT papers that provide some evidence bearing on the question. The lower incidence density of GI infection between 3 and 6 months is the only 'risk' we have documented with 3 versus 6 months of EBF – and that in a setting with very low risks of GI infection – owing to strict hygienic practices, prolonged maternity leaves, and absence of day care under the age of 3 years. Two other areas are worth mentioning, however. First, our statistical power to observe a difference in IQ is limited by the very small numbers of PROBIT women (even in our experimental group) who did EBF for 6 months. (The WHO recommendation at the time PROBIT children were born was EBF for 4–6 months, and that was what our experimental intervention encouraged.)

Second, the protection against SIDS afforded by BF (versus not BF) is quite robust, but information is very limited on whether EBF provides greater protection than partial BF. Given the likely mechanism related to respiratory infection, however, and the peak ages for SIDS risk (2–6 months), it seems plausible to me that EBF for 6 months would be advantageous. I freely admit, however, that this is purely speculation on my part!

Hope this helps, but I'm sure it won't settle the debate.

References

1. Schünemann HJ, Zhang Y, Oxman AD (2019) How to distinguish opinion from evidence in guidelines. *British Medical Journal* 366, l4606.

2. Panda SC (2006) Medicine: science or art? *Mens Sana Monographs* 4, 127–38.

3. Ip S, Chung M, Raman G, *et al.* (2007) Breastfeeding and maternal and infant health outcomes in developed countries. Evidence Report/Technology Assessment No. 153. AHRQ Publication No. 07-E007 April 2007. *Evidence Report Technology Assessment* 153, 1–186.

4. Velle-Forbord V, Skrastad RB, Salvesen O, *et al.* (2019) Breastfeeding and long-term maternal metabolic health in the HUNT study: a longitudinal population-based cohort study. *British Journal of Obstetrics and Gynaecology* 126, 526–34.

5. Der G, Batty D, Deary IJ (2006) Effect of breastfeeding on intelligence in children: prospective study, sibling pairs analysis, and meta-analysis. *British Medical Journal* 4, 333(7575), 945. Available at: https://www.ncbi.nlm.nih.gov/pmc/articles/PMC 1633819/pdf/bmj33300945.pdf (last accessed August 2022).

6. Horta BL, Victora CG (2013) *Long-term effects of breastfeeding. A systematic review. World Health Organization.* Available at: http://apps.who.int/iris/bitstream/handle/ 10665/79198/9789241505307_eng.pdf;jsessionid=FFD92C1D1EFD8158876 D7E831A761C55?sequence=1 (last accessed August 2022).

7. Lucas A, Morley R, Cole TJ, *et al.* (1992) Breast milk and subsequent intelligence quotient in children born preterm. *The Lancet* 339, 261–64.

8. Lucas A, Morley R (1994) Does early nutrition in infants born before term programme later blood pressure? *British Medical Journal* 309, 304–08.

9. Kramer MS, Matush L, Vanilovich I, *et al.* (2009) A randomized breastfeeding promotion intervention did not reduce child obesity in Belarus. *Journal of Nutrition* 139, 417S–21S. DOI: 10.3945/jn.108.097675. Available at: https://pubmed.ncbi. nlm.nih.gov/19106322/?from_term=Martin+RM+bELARUS&from_pos=10 (last accessed August 2022).

10. Yang S, Martin RM, Oken E, *et al.* (2018) Breastfeeding during infancy and neurocognitive function in adolescence: 16-year follow-up of the PROBIT cluster-randomized trial. *PLoS Med* (2015), e1002554. DOI: 10.1371/journal. pmed.1002554. Available at: https://www.ncbi.nlm.nih.gov/pmc/articles/ PMC5909901/ (last accessed August 2022).

11. Kramer MS, Chalmers B, Hodnett ED, *et al.* (2001) Promotion of breastfeeding intervention trial (PROBIT): a randomized trial in the Republic of Belarus. *Journal of the American Medical Association* 285, 413–20. Available at: https://pubmed.ncbi. nlm.nih.gov/11242425/ (last accessed August 2022).

12. Martin RM, Patel R, Kramer MS, *et al.* (2013) Effects of promoting longer-term and exclusive breastfeeding on adiposity and insulin-like growth factor-I at age 11.5 years: a randomized trial. *Journal of the American Medical Association* 309, 1005–13. DOI: 10.1001/jama.2013.167. Available at: https://pubmed.ncbi.nlm.nih.gov/23483175/ (last accessed August 2022).

13. Flohr C, Henderson AJ, Kramer MS, *et al.* (2018) Effect of an intervention to promote breastfeeding on asthma, lung function, and atopic eczema at age 16 years: follow-up of the PROBIT randomized trial. *Journal of the American Medical Association Pediatrics* (1721), e174064. DOI: 10.1001/jamapediatrics.2017.4064. Available at: https://pubmed.ncbi.nlm.nih.gov/29131887/ (last accessed August 2022).

14. Martin RM, Kramer MS, Patel R, *et al.* (2017) Effects of promoting long-term, exclusive breastfeeding on adolescent adiposity, blood pressure, and growth trajectories: a secondary analysis of a randomized clinical trial. *Journal of the American Medical Association Pediatric* 171, e170698. DOI: 10.1001/jamapediatrics.2017.0698.

15. Ballardini N, Kramer MS, Oken E, *et al.* (2019) Associations of atopic dermatitis and asthma with child behaviour: results from the PROBIT cohort. *Clinical and Experimental Allergy* 49, 1235–44. DOI: 10.1111/cea.13417.

16. WHO (2018) *Information note. Clarification on the classification of follow-up formulas for children 6-36 months as breastmilk substitutes.* CC BY-NC-SA 3.0 IGO licence. Available at: https://apps.who.int/iris/bitstream/handle/10665/275875/WHO-NMH-NHD-18.11-eng.pdf?ua=1 (last accessed August 2022).

17. Sankar MJ, Sinha B, Chowdhury R, *et al.* (2015) Optimal breastfeeding practices and infant and child mortality: a systematic review and meta-analysis. *Acta Paediatrica* 104S467), 3–13. DOI:10.1111/apa.13147.

18. Harder T, Bergmann R, Kallischnigg G, Plagemann A (2005) Duration of breastfeeding and risk of overweight: a meta-analysis. *American Journal of Epidemiology* 162, 397–403. DOI:10.1093/aje/kwi222.

19. Azad MB, Nickel NC, Bode L, *et al.* (2021) Breastfeeding and the origins of health: Interdisciplinary perspectives and priorities. *Maternal and Child Nutrition* 17, e13109.

CHAPTER 9

The journey from scientific research to clinical practice

Clinical nutrition research in infancy and childhood has played a pivotal role in establishing relationships between nutrient intake and specific health outcomes. However, there are many challenges and considerations that are unique to early-life nutrition studies, the most critical issue being that it is not possible to undertake a randomized controlled trial (RCT) that compares breastfeeding with formula feeding, because this is correctly considered to be unethical.

An RCT is a study in which a number of similar people are randomly assigned to two (or more) groups to test a specific drug, treatment or other intervention. The intervention (experimental) group receives the intervention being tested; the other group is a comparison or control group which receives an alternative intervention, or a dummy intervention (placebo), or no intervention at all. The only difference between the two groups is that one receives the intervention, and the other does not. In a 'double-blind' RCT, the control group may receive a placebo that is indistinguishable from the intervention, and both the participants and the researchers undertaking the assessments are unaware of who is receiving the intervention. This information is only revealed when the study is complete and data analysis is undertaken. The point of this is to eliminate bias in the results.

Unfortunately this method is not ethically possible in breastfeeding studies. Studying the effect of specific nutrients in the early months of life within an RCT is therefore limited to infants whose parents have decided to formula feed their children. An RCT can be undertaken in which infants are randomized to an intervention formula that includes the nutrient under investigation, or to a control formula without the nutrient (but which is otherwise nutritionally identical to the intervention formula). RCTs can be carried out on infants who are commenced on complementary foods and on the nutrients within those foods.

Observational studies are an alternative, which can be undertaken to compare breastfed and formula-fed children, but these are subject to known and unknown confounding variables that may cause significant bias.

Intervention studies

The potential methodological difficulties of RCTs include the:

- selection of intake levels
- duration of intervention
- measurements of outcomes
- attrition (drop-out or loss) of participants.

Nutrition intervention studies are very different from those that test a new drug to treat conditions such as hypertension. In a new drug study of an antihypertensive, participants will not have been previously exposed to the drug. Levels of the new drug in their blood can be measured and reflect the dose of the drug. Their blood pressure can be measured to determine whether the drug is effective in lowering it. However, in nutrient intervention studies, the participants will have previously received some of the nutrient in their diets before the study, which presents difficulties because the nutrient may be stored in different tissues in the body. Moreover, providing a nutrient that is suspected to be deficient may affect certain aspects of nutritional metabolism that are not identified as an 'outcome measure'; or there may not be a *single* nutrient deficiency so the intervention may not be effective because of deficiencies of other related nutrients. Clinical and functional assessments can be particularly difficult during the early years, therefore to maximize sensitivity of the assessment a large number of participants may be required in both the intervention and control groups, which may impact on recruitment and subsequent attrition.

In the face of challenges like these, it is difficult to achieve a perfect study. Judgement must be made about whether the evidence from a study is 'good enough' to influence practice, to which end there are systems for assessing the strength of evidence and the quality of the methodology. Systematic reviews examine multiple studies on a specific condition and subject the collective data to meta-analysis. Recently systematic reviews of systematic reviews are being carried out and published These can provide a broad perspective of the data, but the strength of the evidence they produce depends on the quality of the *original* data.

In the area of infant feeding, the authors of systematic reviews may report that the assessment of quality is low, or that the original studies were conducted several decades previously. Or it might be that the geographical location of the studies varied markedly. However, as systematic reviews are generally welcomed by editors of journals, they tend to dominate policy decision-making.

To illustrate the many research, clinical, regulatory and political issues that can influence the journey of a specific nutrient from the research arena to its approval for inclusion in infant and young child diets, I now describe what happened with the long-chain polyunsaturated omega-3 fatty acid, docosahexaenoic acid (most commonly referred to as DHA).

Docosahexaenoic acid (DHA)

Although the importance of fatty acids for human health and wellbeing was initially recognized almost ninety years ago,[1] it is only during the last three decades that there has been considerable interest in the roles of long-chain polyunsaturated fatty acids (PUFAs) in infant nutrition, growth and development. The fatty acids that have attracted the greatest interest in infant feeding are DHA and arachidonic acid (ARA) which is an omega-6 fatty acid. The difference between omega-3 and omega-6 relates to their structure, and their function varies.

The seminal work of Manuel Martinez demonstrated the rapid uptake of DHA and ARA by the infant brain during the first 1000 days of life. This has been the driver for many scientists, clinical researchers, nutritionists, developmental psychologists and epidemiologists to contribute to clarifying the roles of these specific fatty acids.[2] The omega-3 and omega-6 fatty acids cannot be synthesized by humans, therefore they are obtained only through the diet. However, DHA and ARA can be synthesized from the shorter chain fatty acids, omega-3 and omega-6 (also known as linoleic acid and alpha-linolenic acid, respectively). This synthesis mechanism is inefficient in early life, and without dietary intake their body levels remain low. Breastmilk *always* contains these two fatty acids, so breastfed infants receive a constant supply during early life. The research has focused on identifying the potential benefits to breastfed infants, and the potential disadvantages to formula-fed infants who do not receive DHA and ARA.

Despite the wealth of information on the functional roles of DHA and ARA from cellular, animal and human studies, and over a thousand publications each year on their role in all aspects of human biology, there is a lack of consensus between policy-makers (with responsibility for infant nutrition) on the specific need for DHA and ARA in early life. The evidence we have predominantly relates to inconsistent findings from a relatively small number of RCTs that have been the subject of four Cochrane systematic reviews. These reviewers have concluded that the quality of data from clinical studies does not allow a recommendation of routine supplementation of full-term infant milk formula with DHA and ARA.[3] Although the studies were rigorously reviewed from an RCT standards perspective, they vary considerably in design, methodology and outcome measures. Moreover, they were all conducted in high-income countries. The evidence base is, therefore, highly selective and may not fully represent the biological importance of DHA and ARA during early or later life. Consequently, current national and international policies may not adequately serve the needs of all infants and children at a time of rapid growth and development.

Cochrane reviews (meta-analyses)

Cochrane reviews are undertaken using the Grading of Recommendations Assessment, Development, and Evaluation (GRADE) system, which rates the quality of evidence and grades the strength of recommendations. There are four levels in the quality assessment:

- *High*—confident that the true effect lies close to the estimate of effect.
- *Moderate*—the true effect is likely to be close to the estimate of effect but may be substantially different.
- *Low*—the true effect may be substantially different from the estimate of effect.
- *Very low*—the true effect is likely to be substantially different from the estimate of effect.

The elements of studies that may influence the strength of evidence include the design and methods, dose–response associations, the magnitude of effect, attrition rates, the risk of bias that may decrease or increase the observed effect, and the estimated overall health gain within the target population. RCTs are generally viewed as high-grade evidence, but the assessment can identify limitations, in the way they were conducted, or weaknesses in certain key domains such as sample size and attrition. Observational studies are generally assumed to provide lower-grade evidence because of the higher risk of bias attributable to a lack of randomization, and the inability of investigators to control for known or unknown confounding factors. However, the strength of observational evidence can be raised by methodological factors, such as large sample size and robust long-term data. With this potential for change in the strength of evidence, it is important to include evidence from all research sources in the assessment process, which is particularly relevant for public health interventions.

Data from randomized clinical trials (RCTs)

The objective of the four Cochrane reviews mentioned above was to assess whether supplementing formula milk with long-chain PUFA is both safe and beneficial for full-term infants.[3] They focused on their effect on visual function, neurodevelopment and physical growth. The limitations of the studies were that they are a small disparate group of studies, demonstrating marked variation in dose and duration of intervention, differences in age at assessment, and there was a diverse range of assessments used. With this level of heterogeneity it was difficult to draw any overall conclusions about the health benefits of long-chain PUFA in early life, other than some evidence of their beneficial effects on visual function and in specific cognitive domains (including problem-solving and attention control).

The heterogeneity of the studies is partly explained by the fact that they were undertaken over a period of two decades and included the very first interventions of DHA and ARA in newborn infants. Understandably, the initial designs and methods reflected a high level of caution, and they did not apply current thinking on doses, duration of the intervention, or choice of assessments. What is surprising is that the DHA and ARA status of the participants wasn't routinely measured at the time of recruitment. As a result, it was not known if there was evidence of deficiency prior to supplementation. Further, all the studies included in the reviews were undertaken in high-income countries, and – on reflection – it is very likely that many of the participants were *not* DHA deficient.[4] This would clearly attenuate the effects of the intervention and, importantly, would conceal any potential benefits in infants with low DHA status.

Appraisal of evidence and the process of making policy

It is important for researchers and policy-makers to distinguish between the appraisal of evidence and the process of making policy. The comment by the reviewers of the Cochrane reviews – that supplementation cannot be rec-ommended based on this RCT data – is an *appraisal* of the evidence, based on systematic review. However, public health interventions are intended to promote or protect health in communities and populations - and their question is - will supplementation of infant formula fed infants provide significant health benefits? So public health policy-making has a broader perspective, one that includes reducing inequality and protecting the most vulnerable. The reported deficiencies in the reviewed RCTs should not only provide learning for researchers and future RCTs, but also provide a marker for policy-makers, as they determine which evidence will provide the best policy on dietary DHA and ARA for vulnerable infants and young children worldwide.

There is a need for new high-quality RCTs to be conducted in appropriate real-world settings, to provide robust information on long-term health outcomes. However, definitive data such as RCTs will not be available for several years. This presents a dilemma for public health policy-makers – do they simply wait for new RCT data to become available or should they, in the meantime, endeavour to protect the interests of infants and young children, especially those living in medium- and low-income countries, by assessing the broader evidence base and developing policies based on reasoned judgement?

What is the best evidence for public health policy-makers?

To increase the value of healthcare services, many countries have established programmes or independent agencies that inform healthcare decision-making through systematically reviewing healthcare interventions (such as the National Institute for Health and Clinical Excellence (NICE) in the UK). In the USA, the AHRQ created the Effective Health Care (EHC) programme in 2005.[5,6] A key element of the programme is a comparative effectiveness review (CER). This aims to determine how the relative benefits and harms of a range of options compare – rather than answering narrow questions on whether a single therapy is safe and effective. As noted in the Cochrane reviews of DHA and ARA, the number of RCTs available to provide direct comparisons is usually relatively small, so there is a risk that the body of evidence is insufficient to draw robust conclusions about benefits and harms. In the most recent Cochrane review (of 2017) the number of selected studies was small and, disappointingly, there were no new cohorts since 2011.[3] In these circumstances, a wider range of opinion from the literature should be sought, including evidence from experimental evidence, placebo-controlled trials and observational studies.

Pragmatism when applying research to practice

The consequences of an inadequate diet, such as deficiencies of DHA and ARA and other key nutrients, are preventable. Therefore, researchers, healthcare workers, policymakers and other key actors, have to carefully consider the level of evidence and decide what actions are appropriate for that strength of evidence.

The transferability of evidence into practice requires multiple factors to be weighed up, such as:

- the perceived magnitude and importance of the problem
- the potential effectiveness and harms of the intervention
- the feasibility of its implementation
- its political acceptability, and
- the public's demand for action.

Different interest groups may advocate for competing recommendations based on the same evidence, but central to the discussion are the dietary needs of the at-risk populations of infants and young children. To make progress a pragmatic approach is required, which may become incremental as further evidence is obtained. To reach agreement on the balance between the level of evidence and the measures required to address need, a framework consisting of several key questions is suggested in Box 9.1.

Box 9.1: An evaluation framework for a pragmatic approach to nutrition policy issues in early life

- Why is a pragmatic approach being considered?
- What is the magnitude of the issue?
- What is the evidence to support a pragmatic dietary intervention in early life?
- What is the intervention, how will it be implemented, and how will the outcomes be measured?
- Is this a cost-effective solution?

Conclusion

There are inherent methodological complexities and ethical considerations that impact on scientific research into infant and young-child nutrition, and translating research into practice can be a tortuous journey. The important mantra in clinical medicine (first and foremost, do no harm) undoubtedly applies to the research and development of nutritional products for infants and children. However, to serve the nutritional needs of this population, key stakeholders must ensure that systems are in place to facilitate an efficient and safe journey from primary-nutrition research to product development, and onward to clinical practice.

This requires the research strategy to be defined, for lessons to be learned from previous studies, and for new methodologies to be robust and effective. To achieve this, the establishment of a Global Research Advisory Centre for infant feeding may improve coordination and increase the level of scrutiny on the product-development process, thus enabling the most promising developments to enter clinical practice within an acceptable timeframe.

Addendum

This chapter is partly based on a previously published article: Forsyth S (2018) Dietary docosahexaenoic acid and arachidonic acid in early life: what is the best evidence for policymakers? *Annals of Nutrition and Metabolism* 72, 210–22.

References

1. Burr GO, Burr MM (1929) A new deficiency disease produced by the rigid exclusion of fat from the diet. *Journal of Biological Chemistry* 82, 345–67.

2. Martinez M (1992) Tissue levels of polyunsaturated fatty acids during early human development. *Journal of Pediatrics* 120, S129–38.

3. Jasani B, Simmer K, Patole SK, Rao SC (2017) Long-chain polyunsaturated fatty acid supplementation in infants born at term (Review). *Cochrane Database of Systematic Reviews* 3, CD000376. DOI: 10.1002/14651858.CD000376.pub4.

4. Forsyth S (2012) Why are we undertaking DHA supplementation studies in infants who are not DHA-deficient? *British Journal of Nutrition* 108, 948.

5. NICE (2022) *NICE Guidance.* Available at: https://www.nice.org.uk/guidance/ (last accessed August 2022).

6. Agency for Healthcare, Research and Quality Effective Healthcare Program (2010) *Methods guide for effectiveness and comparative effectiveness reviews: Selecting observational studies for comparing medical interventions.* Available at: https://www.effectivehealthcare.ahrq.gov/search–for–guides–reviews–and reports/?pageaction–displayProduct&productID=454#1509/ (last accessed August 2022).

CHAPTER 10

Family-friendly policies—
less idealism and more realism

Infant-feeding policies have to be 'family friendly' if they are going to engage effectively with the target population. It is a prerequisite for parents to feel a sense of ownership about the feeding recommendations for their children, without feeling pressurized or confused by the actions of organizations that should be ensuring that infant feeding is an enjoyable and rewarding experience. Unfortunately, infant feeding generates many conflicting opinions in policy and practice, creating confusion and anxiety within families, undermining their confidence and commitment, with an impact on the nutritional care of their children.

Philosophical divisions

Philosophical divisions within infant-feeding policy-making and clinical practice were clearly identified by a study of a cohort of families in Scotland.[1] The aim was to examine the interactions between parents, health professionals, organizations and systems during the period of infant feeding. It was evident that within the extended family and professional network, there were characteristics that allowed interviewees to be classified as idealistic or realistic about infant feeding. The 'idealists', it was noted, were committed to the construct of ideal feeding and were strong advocates of guidelines espousing optimum infant feeding. The 'realists' comprised women, families and (often) health professionals who felt they had to adopt pragmatic measures that were not compliant with the current perceived ideal in order to exist in their *real* world. The study concluded that there is conflict across the idealistic and realistic divide, which generates multiple negative emotions that have an impact on infant-feeding decisions.

It is likely that the seeds of the 'idealism versus realism' paradigm experienced at a family level in Scotland were sown at global-policy level, in Geneva, where philosophical positions also exist. From the direction of emergent global infant-feeding policy, idealism is clearly the dominant force. However, if infant-feeding policy is to be effective and serve the interests of diverse populations worldwide, the currently partisan approach needs to change to a more inclusive process – one that carefully balances the aspirations of idealists with the more fundamental real-life concerns of realists. This requires engagement with all stakeholders – both idealists and realists – and it can be achieved by complying with the core statement of the Code, which:

> *"... affirms the need for governments, organizations of the UN, NGOs, experts in various related disciplines, consumer groups and industry to cooperate in activities that aim to improve maternal, infant and young-child health and nutrition".*[2]

Public engagement

A review of public engagement and policy-making stated that effective policy requires transparency and accessibility and the responsiveness of as wide a range of citizens as possible.[3] To be successful, these elements must relate to all stages of the design and delivery of public services, in order to improve understanding of the evolving and diverse needs of populations. It is also important to reach out beyond the 'usual suspects' and avoid the risk of policy being hijacked by a vociferous few who are unlikely to be representative of the silent majority. Compliance with infant-feeding policy requires consensus from parents – and consensus *from* parents requires consultation *with* parents. As the needs of a population or society evolve, policies have to adapt. One example is the rapid expansion of the female workforce and laws on freedom of information that underline the importance of information access – not only in terms of human rights, but also as a right of good governance.

The Code states that any information provided by manufacturers and distributors to health professionals regarding products within the scope of the Code should be restricted to 'scientific and factual matters'. It is also stated that parents should *only* receive information on formula feeding from health professionals.[2] This restrictive approach to the transmission of information from infant-formula companies contrasts with information that can be made available to parents on breastfeeding, from a wide range of outlets, including advocates, activists and the general media. No restrictions are placed on these sources regarding expressing opinions or offering advice on breastfeeding. Furthermore, with these external sources there is no certainty that any information provided is scientific or factual or not heavily biased. The term 'scientific and factual' is not defined in the Code, so it is open to interpretation and differing personal judgements. As a consequence it is a source of ongoing acrimony and division.

Attempting to restrict the dissemination of information on one aspect of infant feeding – and not on other key elements – can be perceived as introducing bias and discrimination to an area of healthcare that should be open and honest if engagement and compliance are to be achieved. The overall objective should be to ensure that parents are protected from misinformation on both formula feeding and breastfeeding, and to allow them to feel comfortable with their infant-feeding choices.

In contrast to the views of 1981, contemporary thinking may be that parents should be free to discuss matters on infant feeding with any organization that is a key stakeholder for infant-feeding. Then they can reassure themselves that they are receiving information that is valid and not unduly influenced by personal self-interest. All around the world, countries have developed economically over the last forty years, and alongside that there has been significant socioeconomic change; today most of the public has immediate access to electronically delivered information which they use in their professional and personal lives, and they are accustomed to accessing search engines, assimilating information, and making choices. It is extremely important that communication with parents is mature and transparent and reflects contemporary expectations. The statement in the Code, that parents can receive scientific and factual information *only* from healthcare workers, reflects the age of the Code.

Interactions with parents should be bidirectional, whereby they are actively involved in determining the elements of a strategy that specifically require their support and compliance, particularly when it is necessary to establish a middle ground between idealists and realists. Table 10.1 (*overpage*) lists potential views of idealists and realists in the context of infant feeding. Parents may have a greater affinity with one of the categories or they may wish to re-arrange these statements to intuitively reflect their preference for personal guidance.

Completing this, or a similar exercise (the act of parents rearranging the elements in terms of importance and relevance to their family) may highlight the priority of serving the needs of families with different expectations and noting that failure to address these needs will inevitably lead to non-compliance.

Although industry behaviour in relation to violation of the Code is unacceptable (and needs to be corrected), the competing concepts of idealism and realism may be making a more potent and potentially damaging contribution to the acrimony and division across the infant-feeding community. Resolution of these issues is more likely to be achieved through consensus, requiring the wisdom of compromise rather than continuing the current practice of overlaying the whole process with a series of punitive recommendations, sanctions and proposed legislation.

Table 10.1: Perceived idealism and realism in policy-making on infant and child nutrition.

	Idealism	Realism
Breastfeeding	6 months' exclusive breastfeeding	4–6 months' exclusive breastfeeding
	2 years' or beyond continuous breastfeeding	1 year or beyond continuous breastfeeding
	Complementary foods from 6 months	Complementary foods from 4–6 months
	Breastmilk substitutes up to 3 years	Breastmilk substitutes up to 1 year
Complementary feeding	Home prepared local foods	Availability of commercial products
Policies	Policies global one-size-fits-all	Policies sensitive to national/family needs
Access to industry	No parental access to formula industry	Access to industry for information
	Health access for scientific and factual matters	Access for exploratory discussions
	No collaborative research with formula industry	Collaboration subject to agreed regulations
	No sponsorship from formula industry	Sponsorship subject to agreed regulations

In courts of law, verdicts are decided by a lay jury, who considers the arguments from the prosecution and the defence. In this analogy, it may be valuable to reflect on what a lay jury comprising parents would conclude from the evidence of the last four decades of conflict between WHO and the infant-formula industry. For example, would they:

- appreciate the benefits of breastfeeding but not agree with the one-size-fits-all approach to the inflexible micromanagement of exclusive and continuing breastfeeding?
- see the importance of the availability of a safe alternative (if required)?
- consider that the revised definition of a breastmilk substitute is problematic?
- believe that current WHO policies on infant nutrition are too idealistic or too realistic (or neither)?

The views of parents are paramount and it needs to be appreciated that listening to, and learning from parents, is a key element of policy development, and if the parental view is distant from that of policy-makers, then non-compliance is inevitable. If the policy-maker response to parental non-compliance is denial and rejection, then division is inevitable. If division becomes entrenched, parental disengagement and self-practice become the norm. If policy-makers do not like the norm, a new cycle of fruitless policy-making begins.

Economic status

The economic status of a country, and that of individual families, is a strong determinant of choice when it comes to infant feeding. This is something that needs to be acknowledged by policy-makers in their policies.[4] With changes in economic status, there is likely to be a shift in infant-feeding patterns that is driven by perceived changes in family priorities. This is represented schematically in Table 10.2.

Table 10.2: Trends in infant-feeding and childhood morbidity and mortality according to global economic status.

	Low-income countries	Emerging economies	High-income countries
Breastfeeding	Prolonged (the primary source of nutrition in early life)	Prevalence reduces to a new steady state	Low prevalence, but evidence of increased initiation and exclusivity
Infant formula	Availability remains relatively low	Rapid increase in sales	High levels of sales reduce
Complementary feeding	Inadequate supplies locally and commercially	Increase in availability	Greater range of commercial options
Nutrition-related morbidity and mortality	Rates of malnutrition, stunting and nutrition-related deaths are high	Rapidly falling mortality, but increase in overweightness and obesity	Low mortality and initial increase in overweightness and obesity now levelling

Historical evidence of socioeconomic change and the impact that it has on infant-feeding practice should be at the heart of future policy-making. Lives and livelihood are inherently linked, which is evident when there is a transition from the poverty-driven passive acceptance of adversity to a situation in which there is a growing sense of social and financial independence in an emerging economy. It is not surprising that, as the lives of a population change, their perspective of infant feeding also changes. In the past, this has manifested through a lower prevalence of breastfeeding and a greater use of infant formula – at least initially.

Evidence from high-income countries suggests that there may be an element of 'rebound', but the current extreme expectations of policy-makers and activist groups are unlikely to be met. Policymakers should not ignore the effects of global movements in economic status and the potential impact that they may have on infant-feeding practice. A key message should be that a global didactic approach will not succeed in the new world of self-determination.

As populations move from a position of poverty and passive acceptance to a new era of opportunity and self-determination, new attitudes and behaviours will influence decisions at the family level. The choice and practice of infant feeding will be considered within a broader family context. It has been suggested that measures should be taken to reverse the trend for increased infant-formula consumption in emerging economies,[4] but with reports of rapidly falling infant and young child mortality in these countries, consideration must focus on the *totality* of factors that influence morbidity and mortality. Therefore, there must be 'new thinking' on the way infant-feeding policy-making more effectively aligns with the accompanying global socioeconomic changes, to achieve an overall health benefit.

The direction of travel adopted by policy-makers should be to pursue the potential benefits of socioeconomic change on the health and wellbeing of infants and young children, bearing in mind how infant-feeding policies can complement such changes. The focus should shift from less rigidity about the timings of breastfeeding and other transitions, to formulating the best combination of health interventions and thus address continuing undernutrition and overnutrition, and the double burden of malnutrition. A health analysis of WHO recommendations should be considered in the context of local circumstances. For example, in more affluent populations it may be pertinent to relax the duration of continuing breastfeeding during the second and third years of life, to place greater emphasis on commencing breastfeeding at birth, thus providing greater breastmilk coverage over the first year of life (the period during which the benefits of breastfeeding have been most clearly documented).

With due diligence to global principles, this should be the role and responsibility of individual regions and countries. They should assess their own level of nutritional risk, and shape infant-feeding policies to meet the broader health and social needs of families at risk. How this flexibility is managed needs to be carefully considered by all stakeholders, at both national and global levels.

And should there be a minimum standard for infant-feeding practice that can be adjusted according to specific national risk factors? A potential stepwise approach to infant-feeding decision-making may be viewed as more realistic and acceptable to parents who are sceptical about being given the same advice if they live in Switzerland or Sierra Leone. It seems obvious that parents should be given information that is relevant to them.

Misleading information

It is vitally important that at all points in the dissemination of information, parents are provided with information that is realistic and balanced – and this especially applies to breastfeeding, infant formula and complementary feeding. Misleading parents with comments and interpretations that fail to provide accurate, pragmatic and verifiable messages about infant feeding must be avoided. Hitherto, this approach was focused on infant-formula companies, but the same level of scrutiny should be applied to all aspects of the infant diet. For example, enthusiasm and commitment to breastfeeding should not result in over-interpretation of data; and a balanced and sensible view of the strengths and limitations of breastfeeding data should be clearly presented.

A common route for disseminating information is through the publication of articles in scientific journals. These may be picked up by journalists and widely spread through various media outlets. One article that has been very extensively referred to in recent years is that by Professor Victora and his colleagues. It was published in *The Lancet Breastfeeding Series* in 2016 and attracted widespread media interest. The headline message was that universal scaling up of breastfeeding to recommended levels will prevent 823,000 deaths annually in children aged below 5 years of age worldwide.[5] This statement now appears to lead on most articles about infant feeding, and it is frequently reiterated by WHO.

The Victora paper is widely referenced as evidence of the importance of breastfeeding and associated health outcomes. However, the content also highlights the difficulties of undertaking retrospective reviews of studies of infant-feeding practice and subsequent outcome measures. Potential limitations of the Victora paper are the gaps in the availability of high-quality data, the complexities of comparing low- and medium-income countries with more affluent nations, and the lack of recognition of the interdependence between breastmilk and complementary foods, or their combined roles in enabling the best health outcome measures.

Further, this intervention was commissioned by WHO, who received sponsorship from the Bill & Melinda Gates Foundation. The objective appears to have been to clarify the extent of the scientific evidence available to support the current WHO global recommendation on infant-feeding policy, with the focus primarily on breastfeeding.

The message from *The Lancet* paper that caught the interest of the media – and therefore parents – was that by scaling up breastfeeding worldwide, 823,000 children's lives will be saved annually. This is now a soundbite for the promotion of breastfeeding, and it usually appears in the first paragraph of any document that relates to breastfeeding. It is, therefore, very important for parents to have some understanding of how the researchers came to their conclusion, so they can be reassured that this is a realistic and balanced message for all families worldwide. In order to achieve this, it is important for the information for parents to meet agreed standards of evidence, for the message to be balanced and transparent, and (as with the standards required for submission to scientific journals) for it to reflect the strengths and limitations of the scientific evidence.

The figure of 823,000 emerges from the text, and although there are supporting documents, the way in which this widely quoted figure has been calculated should be explained in a way that is appropriate for parents to comprehend – as well as for those who are disseminating this information. The Lives Saved Tool (LiST) is a software package that has been developed over the past ten years with the aim of estimating the impact that scaling up community-based interventions would have on under-five years mortality (see the correspondence from Professor Victora in Box 10.1 (in the *Addendum* to this chapter).

Understanding the methodology is a very important starting point for readers, for which more clarity is required. For example, there were issues regarding the quality of the breastfeeding data, with limited information on breastfeeding rates from high-income countries, derived from only twenty-seven out of thirty-five countries. And there are differences in the way the data were categorized. Also, there were long intervals between the breastfeeding period and the point at which parents recalled the information. The authors used other sources of information to try and fill gaps and, where they considered it necessary, they estimated the proportion of infants breastfed at twelve months of age on the basis of information available for breastfeeding at six months of age (and vice versa).

The rates of breastfeeding in low- and middle-income countries were more complete, although the distinction between exclusive and predominant breastfeeding was frequently unclear and therefore this is undoubtedly a weakness of this study and also raises questions about the robustness of data that is used to support WHO policy on exclusive breastfeeding. It is evident that because of the lack of clarity between exclusive and predominant breastfeeding the key analysis was a comparison of partial breastfeeding versus no breastfeeding with the definition of partial breastfeeding used by Victora and colleagues being:

> *"Breastmilk from mother or wet nurse or expressed breast milk, and any other liquids or non-liquids, including both milk and non-milk products".*

Because of the lack of published data on complementary foods, complementary feeding was not included in the analysis, which significantly impacts on the validity and credibility of their analysis because complementary feeding is a vital component of the infant diet and plays a key role in determining growth, health and development from six months of age. Without including complementary foods, the analysis is based on an infant-feeding regimen that does not – and never will – reflect infant-feeding policy in any country worldwide.

There is yet another problem. The authors stated that they used the LiST to predict how many deaths of children below the age of 5 years would be prevented if breastfeeding patterns were scaled up in the seventy-five countries with the highest child death rates, commenting that these countries account for 95% of such deaths worldwide. This statement indicates that the remaining 122 countries in the world only accounted for 5% of the under-5 years deaths, and this again raises the issue of the appropriateness of a one-size-fits-all global infant-feeding policy. Clearly this analysis is relevant to the countries whose data were utilized in the analysis but translating it to the environment of affluent countries – in which child mortality is low, death from infection is significantly reduced, breastfeeding rates are low, complementary feeding is more readily available, and housing and living circumstances are markedly different – raises questions about the validity of this approach. There is no data on morbidity, and it needs to be underlined that breastfeeding alone will not prevent malnutrition, wasting and stunting, and therefore an unfortunate but more accurate headline may be that in those circumstances breastfeeding is delaying death and what these families need is life-saving food. The outcome data are entirely dependent on the quality of the original data that was analyzed. When there are significant differences in the quality and quantity of data between high and low-income countries, the rearrangement, reclassification and readjustment of the data does not fully address the issues of absent or incomplete data.

This leads to speculation about the statement of 823,000 lives saved. And what does this mean for individual countries? The paper does not provide an international breakdown of the number of lives saved. The original data were obtained from countries with the highest child mortality rates, so it is clearly of some relevance to them, but how should high-income countries respond? Would it not have been more helpful if the data collection and analysis had been considered at the levels of high- middle-, and low-income countries? In so doing, the most appropriate infant-feeding categories could have been considered for each income level. For example, there seems to be little point in looking at the health effects of prolonged breastfeeding (for over a year) in high-income countries when most countries do not collect this data. The desire of WHO to take a global perspective on infant feeding and attempt to have a global policy, global target and global data-collection standards may be attractive in theory, but *only* if the data meets acceptable standards of quality and quantity. Attempting to fill gaps in knowledge by adjusting for the many variables in demography, socioeconomic status, nutrition and healthcare, and many other confounders, inevitably provides data that will be assessed as low quality. A more pragmatic approach would involve a focus on specific countries and communities, collecting and analyzing their own data, and setting their own infant-feeding policies – it might provide a more reliable and robust way forward.

In the past, Victora and colleagues tended to interpret their data with far more caution, as evidenced in their 2013 assessment (this is described in detail in Chapter 8). The number of new publications since 2013 is relatively few, so there needs to be a clear justification for adopting a different viewpoint.

Interestingly, I studied their 2016 publication more thoroughly, a year after publication, and there appeared to be errors in the supplementary material they provided. I contacted Professor Victora and received a prompt reply (see the *Addendum* to this chapter). We were both of the view that, despite the extensive interest in the publication, it is very surprising that the errors hadn't been identified beforehand, particularly by his co-authors, who included two members of WHO. Victora was confident however, that the errors did not influence the outcome of the study. He also commented on the absence of data on complementary feeding and also expressed the concern that many of the studies provided used 'old' data, and that their relevance to societies in both developed and developing countries may differ markedly. His comment about researchers appearing to be less interested in this area of investigation was also significant. This is referred to elsewhere in this critique, and undoubtedly the internal politics within the infant-feeding community is a disincentive.

Finally, if you enter the phrase '823,000 lives saved' into a search engine like Google, you will get many pages of websites quoting it, including some from WHO, UNICEF, Save the Children Fund and many media outlets, as well as numerous personal blogs. None are accompanied by information on the potential strengths and limitations of the research. It is important that leading health organizations should ensure that messages from scientific papers are accurately and responsibly interpreted on their websites, and it is advised that these organizations read the whole of the original paper and any supplementary data. Their responsibility is to highlight to the general public exactly what the authors are saying and (arguably more importantly) what they are not saying. By so doing they maintain their neutrality rather than become a source of bias and self-interest.

The importance of choosing the right language

It is not only important to ensure that the content of communications is accurate and unable to be misrepresented, but the language used to communicate needs to be appropriate, for example with families. It is ironic that so much of the controversy about infant feeding revolves around the term 'breastmilk substitutes', a term that was created by policy-makers but is ignored by parents and health professionals. In the past, the key foods for infants were clearly understood to be breastmilk, infant formula and solid foods, and these continue to be the terms that are used by parents. The term 'weaning' was replaced by 'complementary feeding' because policy-makers felt that weaning indicated that mothers should gradually reduce breastfeeding, whereas they preferred the concept that solid foods should be seen as *complementing* breastmilk. This situation has been complicated by WHO, who state that all milk products marketed for children up to the age of three years should be considered to be 'breastmilk substitutes', sparking a debate about whether liquid nutritional products consumed during the third year of life should be called breastmilk substitutes, or complementary foods, or simply drinks.[6] The argument put forward by WHO is that even in the third year of life, it is important that the increase in the food component of the diet (liquid and solid) *complements* rather than replaces breastmilk.

A fundamental problem is the misrepresentation of the term 'complementary' feeding. The mistake is the assumption that this should refer to all fluids and solids that complement breastmilk, but it would make more sense if the concept referred to *all* components of the infant and young-child diet complementing each other. This would bring a focus to the importance of the child diet being nutritionally balanced, and for the nutritional components of the diet to evolve as the child grows and develops. Such a distinction may help defuse the esoteric argument about whether complementary foods are displacing, replacing or complementing breastmilk – and hopefully reduce the acrimony and division that has been generated. The breastfeeding special-interest groups will be concerned that this devalues breastfeeding, but the approach may more clearly demonstrate the importance of the interdependence of the key foods in early life – including breastmilk. This theme, of the different foods complementing each other, may be useful for developing nutrition regimens for both severe and moderate malnutrition, and reduce the risk of double burden of malnutrition.

Without precise measures, in practice it is difficult to determine whether drinks or food complement or replace breastmilk, however, as previously noted, breastfed children in developing countries have an average breastmilk energy intake (according to WHO/UNICEF, 1998) that declines with age (Table 10.3). There is a similar pattern with the average intakes of breastfed children in industrialized countries (WHO/UNICEF, 1998).[7]

Table 10.3: Comparison of average energy intakes from breastmilk in breastfed children in developing and industrialized countries (WHO/UNICEF, 1998).[7]

Age	Developing countries	Industrialized countries
6–8 months	413 kcal/day	486 kcal/day
9–11 months	379 kcal/day	375 kcal/day
12–23 months	346 kcal/day	313 kcal/day

With this established trend of reducing breastmilk intake with age, it can be assumed that intake will reduce further during the third year of life.[7] This decline is to be expected as the need for solid foods with a higher nutritional value than breastmilk is required to meet the increasing needs of the rapidly growing and developing child. Theoretically, to substantiate WHO's assertion that other milk-related products should not replace breastmilk during the complementary feeding period, mothers would need to continue to provide the daily volume of breastmilk that they achieved at the end of the six-months' exclusive breastfeeding period, which would require them to continue breastfeeding around five to six times a day, with the infant consuming approximately 1000 ml of breastmilk daily until the age of three years. Where is the evidence that this daily volume of breastmilk provides additional benefit to an infant? Alternatively, because of breastmilk's low energy and nutrient density compared to complementary foods, caution is required in order to prevent a potential negative effect on growth and development.

The Code[2] defined complementary foods as:

> *"… any food, whether manufactured or locally prepared, suitable as a complement to breastmilk or to infant formula, when either become insufficient to satisfy the nutritional requirements of the infant".*

This interpretation of complementary food makes sense with respect to the infancy period (from birth to twelve months), which as previously argued appears to have been the original time period considered by WHO's executive board when presenting the Code to the WHA. But for the young-child period (one to three years) it appears misplaced. In this time, the priority is to establish a diversified diet that will meet the child's nutritional requirements and transition into a nutritious family diet. It seems that WHO is more concerned about the possibility that the liquid component of the child diet at this time will displace breastmilk, and therefore WHO states that these liquids should be understood to be breastmilk substitutes (discussed in more detail in Chapter 7). The likelihood is that most parents will consider this discussion on displacing breastmilk by other liquids and foods at the age of three years as unnecessarily abstruse, driven by self-interest, and an unnecessary diversion from the real issues relating to childhood nutrition both locally and worldwide. Moreover, they will probably take a more pragmatic view and simply see this stage in their child's feeding development as a gradual transition to a young-child's diet and onwards to a family diet in which all foods complement each other to provide a healthy diet.

Advising on policy

The Code recognizes that all infants are not breastfed, and some are only partially breastfed. Therefore there is a need for infant formulas to provide a safety net for the infant. In these circumstances it is important that the composition of the formula represents the best scientific evidence and allows the infant to receive the best alternative to breastmilk. Standards for the composition of infant formulas have been set by organizations such as Codex Alimentarius, the European Food Safety Authority, and the Food and Drug Administration, but this is a process that can be challenging. Traditional divisions tend to open up, whereby WHO and breastfeeding interest groups are reluctant to allow the inclusion of new nutritional factors (such as long chain polyunsaturated fatty acids, oligosaccharides, pre- and probiotics), on the grounds that they believe evidence of benefit to be lacking, so adding them to formulas simply increases sales and profits for the formula industry.

This is where it would be helpful to have an independent view, but it presents the dilemma of who can be considered by all stakeholders to be independent and to have the knowledge and expertise to make a balanced and informed judgement. WHO takes the view that such an individual should not have ties with industry. This would rule out researchers and clinicians who have experience of undertaking clinical intervention feeding studies in infants, as they now have to be conducted in collaboration with industry if the intervention product is to meet nutrition and safety standards. Parents are likely to take the view that they want all relevant researchers, clinicians and policy-makers to collectively advise and agree on the best policy for their infants and young children. They may question why those advising them on the best infant formula are not working closely with industry to ensure that the products reflect the best science, address the diverse clinical needs of infants and young children, and are marketed appropriately. Parents expect all health-related professionals to be responsible and transparent, including WHO officials. And if parents have concerns, they need to have guidance on how to raise issues with the relevant regulatory body for the relevant stakeholder. Of the current stakeholders, healthcare has well-documented channels through which parents and others can submit complaints regarding alleged substandard care or professional conduct, however this is less clear for other stakeholders. Governance and regulation are discussed further in Chapter 14.

Equality, caring and respect

Throughout the Covid-19 pandemic there were numerous examples of personal tragedies relating to health and social care of families, with the most vulnerable people resorting to measures that for many would have been unthinkable in normal times. In the UK, an infant-feeding matter that attracted considerable interest was the availability of infant formulas at food banks. Views expressed on the issue were clearly divided –breastfeeding interest groups were strongly against food banks providing infant formula, and the more socially sensitive organizations supported the option for food banks to have infant formula available for emergency situations.[8–10] In their information sheet, UNICEF UK stated this seemed like a practical solution, but carried a risk and the potential to cause harm, so they did not support food-bank staff handing out infant formula. Their advice was for all local authorities to have a clear pathway for the distribution of infant formula as part of the local authority emergency-food provision system, and for food banks to put in place robust referral systems.[8] The UNICEF UK proposal was robustly challenged by FEED,[9] a Scotland-based charity set up by a group of mothers to support mothers. This conflict of opinion was considered in an article published in the *British Medical Journal* under the title 'Food banks and infant formula: who knows best?'.[10]

It is important such issues are considered not only from organizational, political and potentially self-interest perspectives, but also from a position that provides a clear understanding of the implications for parents who find themselves in this difficult situation. In the midst of the pandemic, social and health services were stretched beyond their limits, and accessing advice from these authorities at that time was not straightforward. Moreover, UNICEF UK included contact details for five global breastfeeding organizations which, to many, appears to be incredibly insensitive and will only succeed in humiliating mothers. There was also an element of discrimination and inequality, in that mothers who had money would be able to go to their local supermarket, take a tin of infant formula from the shelf without needing anyone to give them advice about formulas, then simply pay at the checkout and feed their baby. It seems that UNICEF UK believes mothers who attend food banks do not know which formula their baby requires, nor that the staff will be able to give advice. The worst possible outcome from this scenario would be that the mother leaves the food bank without formula for her infant and with the risk of potential harm to infant and possibly mother, who would be held accountable?

There is a long history of adults behaving badly over infant nutrition and this scenario encapsulates some behaviours that are evident in the wider infant-feeding policy-making process. It is difficult not to surmise that UNICEF UK's rather bureaucratic approach to this personal infant-feeding crisis, and the decision not to provide infant formula in emergency situations in food banks, is at least partially driven by their overriding commitment to breastfeeding and their antipathy towards infant-formula companies. Whereas the more socially sensitive organizations, such as FEED, recognize the need to actively support mothers in the most dire circumstances and to respect their decisions on formula feeding, underlining the need to provide them with an interim supply of formula to prevent potentially serious complications from lack of fluid and nutrition, and ensuring ongoing support is available if required.[9] The article in the *British Medical Journal* asked the question – *who knows best*? This answer is – the person who *cares the most*.

Interface with health professionals

A key determinant of infant-feeding policy should be the relationship between parents and health professionals, but this is underappreciated by policy-makers. A continuing concern for parents is that they see global decisions being made by people they do not know and in places that are far removed from their own circumstances. Despite these factors there is an assumption that parents will blindly comply. Parents have more faith in their health professionals, and they believe that they will provide them with the best advice for their children. It is important for health professionals to consider infant nutritional concerns in the context of WHO's recommendations, but also to make clinical decisions based on their clinical judgement. Therefore, inevitably, on occasions their advice may not align with that of WHO, but this should not be interpreted by policy-makers or lay organizations as an example of non-compliance. These are examples of health professionals responding to needs of individual infants and their families by providing personalized clinical care that cannot be regulated by population-based global recommendations.

Infant-feeding practice is not an exact science, so a 'robotic' approach to policy-making should be resisted. It is important that the relationship between health professionals and parents allows for open and constructive discussions that culminate in an infant-feeding plan which meets the needs of the child and family. From a pragmatic point of view, this may not include the precise timings of exclusive breastfeeding for exactly six months, or the introduction of complementary foods at exactly six months, or continuing breastfeeding for two years or beyond. What is most important is that the nutritional regimen meets the needs of the individual child, and that their parents are able to enjoy the rewarding experience of feeding and bonding with their child. Critically, feelings of guilt and shame associated with failing to comply with an inflexible WHO global breastfeeding policy must be avoided.

Conclusion

Policies for infant and young-child feeding should be family friendly. A key element of this should be the relationship between parents and their health professionals. Policy-makers have to appreciate the importance of this relationship and respect the need for a partnership that is sensitive to the needs of each individual child. Policy-makers also need to ensure that the information made available to parents is relevant, pragmatic and verifiable. In truth, some of the best ideas can emerge from parents, and the blue-sky thinking of WHO and their colleagues in breastfeeding-interest groups must align more closely with the grass-roots realism of families and their health professionals. A key outcome of this process should be that policy-making becomes less polarized, less rigid, and more individualized and more caring.

Addendum

I wrote to Professor Victora following the publication of his article in The Lancet in 2016 regarding the occurrence of errors in the supplementary material and to clarify other aspects of the study. His response came quickly and is reproduced here with his permission (Box 10.1). Note, the following acronyms were used in these letters: BF for breastfeeding, DHS for demographic and health surveys, MICS for multiple indicator cluster surveys, and RR for relative risk.

Box 10.1: Personal correspondence with Professor Victora following publication of his article in *The Lancet Breastfeeding Series* (2016)

Letter to Professor Victora (20 December 2017)

Your Lancet paper has attracted considerable interest and, in particular, the headline statement that scaling-up breastfeeding to a near-universal level could prevent 823,000 annual deaths in children younger than 5 years. It is with regard to this aspect of your paper that I contact you. I have carefully read the paper and the supporting information, and I would be grateful for clarification on the following.

First, you state that the relative risks for the protection against all infectious causes of death were obtained from your new meta-analyses (Sankar et al., 2015), however I note that the studies selected for the analysis are not recent and the median for the year of publication of the 13 studies is 1994, with the first publication in 1987 and the most recent 2006. For the host countries involved in these studies there have been significant improvements (approximately 65% reduction) in child mortality over the last 30 years and I therefore ask if applying the relative risks relating to breastfeeding practices, which were calculated when mortality rates were 2–3-fold higher than your baseline year of 2013, have an impact on the calculation of present-day preventable deaths? Second, in the supporting information [in one of the tables] scaled rates of breastfeeding by age of child is confusing as it appears to indicate that the scaling-up included exclusive breastfeeding from 6–24 months. Is this correct?

Third, in the main text, reference is made to WHO breastfeeding goals, including a target of 90% for any breastfeeding from 6–23 months, and you note that five countries already have levels that are above this target - Nepal, Rwanda, Ethiopia, Burundi and Guinea. However, these countries have extremely high levels of under-5 mortality (mean 56 per 1000 live births) and an extremely high prevalence of stunting (mean 44% of children under the age of 5 years). The data underline the importance of breastfeeding being adequately complemented by safe and nutritious complementary foods. I wondered why you did not consider the scaling-up of complementary feeding in your study and provide estimates of the effect that this has on infant and child mortality. Clearly, breastfeeding and complementary feeding are interdependent, and the balance of this interdependency changes during the first 2 years of life as the nutritional contribution of complementary feeding becomes more critical. Focusing entirely on breastfeeding appears to be inappropriately restrictive and, without data relating to complementary feeding, the breastfeeding data may be misleading. I would welcome your comments.

Response from Professor Victora (21 December 2017)

Many thanks for your interest in our Lancet paper. You raise some important issues, and here is my response. First, you are right that the papers on BF and mortality risk are quite old. Unfortunately, there is nothing we can do about it, as we did a thorough search of the literature, and it seems that the interest in this topic has waned since the 1990s. To avoid the problem that you mention (changes in levels and causes of death in recent years), we derived cause-specific relative risks of mortality from the old studies and used the Lives Saved Tool (LiST) to apply these RRs to the current distribution of causes of death in low- and middle-income countries. We believe that this is a satisfactory solution to estimating deaths prevented. Second, thanks for spotting the mistake in [one of the tables]. We modelled the impact of partial (not exclusive) BF rates of 90% from 6–24 months. Amazing that we did not spot this mistake earlier, nor any of our readers as far as we know! By the way, [another table] is also wrong as the reference group (RR of 1.0) should be partial BF, not exclusive BF, and the RR of 2.09 should apply to no BF [versus] partial [BF]. This is a bit embarrassing.

Thirdly, I fully agree with you that the issue of the quality of complementary foods is very important, and it may explain why countries high long durations of BF – 24 months or longer – still present high mortality rates. I would argue that their mortality rates would be even higher in the absence of BF, but I take your point on the need to consider the quality, variety and frequency of complementary foods. While planning The Lancet series, we discussed this extensively, but in the end The Lancet only allowed us two papers with up to 5000 words each, and there was no way we could also cover complementary feeding. We also looked at the extent of existing data on complementary feeding and found that such information has only been recently incorporated in surveys such as DHS and MICS, and we concluded that there was not sufficient information to model the impact of complementary feeding. The data availability situation is changing rapidly, so that in the near future there may be enough information on this topic.

I hope that I have addressed the issues you have raised - even if I don't have the final answers to some of these.

References

1. Hoddinott P, Craig LCA, Britten J, *et al.* (2012) A serial qualitative interview study of infant feeding experiences. *BMJ Open* 2, e000504. Available at: DOI:10.1136/ https://bmjopen.bmj.com/content/bmjopen/2/2/e000504.full.pdf/ (last accessed August 2022).

2. WHO (1981) *International Code of Marketing of Breastmilk Substitutes.* Available at: https://apps.who.int/iris/bitstream/handle/10665/40382/9241541601.pdf? sequence=1&isAllowed=y (last accessed August 2022).

3. OECD (2009) *Focus on citizens: Public engagement for better policy and services.* Available at: http://www.oecd.org/governance/regulatorypolicy/focusoncitizens publicengagementforbetterpolicyandservices.htm (last accessed August 2022).

4. Neves PAR, Gatica-Domínguez G, Rollins NC, *et al.* (2020) Infant formula consumption is positively correlated with wealth, within and between countries: a multi-country study. *Journal of Nutrition* 150, 910–17.

5. Victora CG, Bahl R, Barros AJD, *et al.* (2016) Breastfeeding in the 21st century: epidemiology, mechanisms, and lifelong effect. *The Lancet* 38, 475–90.

6. Forsyth S (2018) Is WHO creating unnecessary confusion over breastmilk substitutes? *Journal of Pediatric Gastroenterology and Nutrition* 67, 760–62.

7. WHO (1998) *Complementary feeding of young children in developing countries: a review of current scientific knowledge.* Available at: https://apps.who.int/iris/handle/10665/65932 (last accessed August 2022).

8. UNICEF Baby Friendly Initiative (2020) *UNICEF UK infosheet: the provision of infant formula at food banks* (updated November 2020). Available at: https://www.unicef.org.uk/babyfriendly/wp–content/uploads/sites/2/2019/05/Provision–of–formula–milk–at–food–banks–Unicef–UK–Baby–Friendly–Initiative.pdf (last accessed August 2022).

9. FEED (2020) *The provision of infant formula at food banks in the UK.* Available at: https://static1.squarespace.com/static/5efa4a95af311446a53c8cab/t/5fd0990c5347e801a823f769/1607506207266/Feed+report+on+formula+at+foodbanks+–+December+9th+2020.pdf (last accessed August 2022).

10. Wise J (2020) Food banks and infant formula: who knows best? *British Medical Journal* 371, m4449.

The relationship of breastfeeding to maternal health

Breastfeeding is reported to provide significant health benefits for mothers as well as their infants. The benefits for mothers include early postnatal weight loss, delayed menstruation and fertility, a reduced risk of obesity, cardiovascular disease and diabetes, and protection against cancer of the breast and ovary.[1] In the majority of these conditions the relationship with breastfeeding is described as an association – a direct causal effect has not been fully established. However, it is important that these associations have been identified and they should be investigated further to establish potential and viable mechanisms to explain the link, and thus provide prospective parents with scientifically robust information.

Breastfeeding, menstruation and infertility

These relationships have attracted attention for some time because of the possibility that breastfeeding may act as a method of birth control, especially in countries in which other methods are not available or acceptable – in fact, this is the best example of a causal effect of breastfeeding that is substantiated by reliable scientific evidence. The data demonstrate that duration of lactation and the duration of infertility are directly related to the suckling pattern of an infant.[2] Stimulation of the nipple during suckling results in three hormonal responses:

- the release of oxytocin from the posterior pituitary to release milk from the breast
- the release of prolactin from the anterior pituitary, which is essential for milk production for subsequent feeds
- the suppression of gonadotrophin from the hypothalamus, which suppresses activity of the ovaries.

During the period of lactational amenorrhoea (the gap in menstruation), secretion of oestradiol by the dominant follicles of the ovary is low leading to low plasma concentrations, in contrast to the increase seen during the follicular phase of the normal menstrual cycle. This suggests there is minimal ovarian activity, as follicular development during the normal cycle is always associated with increased oestrogen secretion. During early lactation (up to 12 weeks post-partum), ultrasound visualization of the ovary shows an absence of follicle development, but at later stages the follicles do develop but oestrogen secretion remains low. The reason is that suckling reduces the secretion of the gonadotrophins known as luteinizing hormone (LH) and follicle-stimulating hormone (FSH).

The established pattern of suckling varies considerably as it is dependent on both the mother and the infant. When suckling is maintained at a high level, ovarian secretion of steroid hormones may be suppressed for several months, sometimes years, even in well-nourished Western societies. When the frequency of suckling is lower, ovarian activity resumes earlier. To maintain amenorrhoea, it has been suggested that the frequency of suckling should be maintained at above five times a day, for a total duration of more than sixty-five minutes a day. Note that these empirical criteria can vary across different populations and therefore are not totally reliable.

The duration of amenorrhoea tends to correlate with the duration of breastfeeding, which may be beneficial in some countries and societies in which other alternatives to birth control are not available, but for a large part of the global population this may be perceived as restricting family-planning options, especially if WHO expects mothers to breastfeed during the child's third year of life. Changes in modern-day living include greater opportunities for women to aspire to further education and career development, and this is reflected by the many women who choose to delay the timing of their first birth. This is clearly a matter for individual national governments, and something that which WHO should reflect on when advising on their global breastfeeding policy.

Breastfeeding, obesity, cardiovascular disease and diabetes

Cardiovascular disease is the leading cause of death among women in developed nations, and obesity is the most common medical condition in women of reproductive age. Type 2 diabetes is a significant complication of obesity, and this triad of disease – cardiovascular, diabetes and obesity – is referred to as 'metabolic syndrome'. Many factors contribute to these conditions and there are suggestions that their prevalence may be reduced in women with a history of breastfeeding. Furthermore, there are many confounding factors that may overlap with these conditions, including the decision to breastfeed. For these reasons, in observational studies, which lack specificity, there is uncertainty about the relation between these conditions and breastfeeding.

Schwarz and colleague, who have been very active in this field, acknowledge the methodological difficulties of conducting such studies.[3-6] In one study, conducted in the US, they recorded various anthropometric measurements and undertook CT scans for visceral obesity (a good predictor of cardiovascular risk) in women aged 46–58 years. They related measurements of adiposity to the women's breastfeeding histories and concluded that pre- or early perimenopausal women who do not breastfeed each of their children for at least three months are significantly more likely to be burdened by visceral fat, and this may increase their risk of an adverse cardiovascular outcome. Despite being one of the more thorough studies of the relationship between breastfeeding, later obesity and cardiovascular risk, the authors discuss extensively the difficulties of undertaking these studies and how such issues might relate to their own study.[3]

> *"Our findings must be interpreted with the understanding that all observational studies may be subject to residual confounding. In this study, duration of breastfeeding was self-reported. Recall or reporting bias may have led to some misclassification of women's breastfeeding history. Prior research has found that women with shorter durations of breastfeeding tended to over-report, while women with longer durations tended to under-report. In addition, the measure of breastfeeding used in this study does not allow estimation of the intensity or exclusivity with which women breastfed their infants. It is possible that more powerful effects would be seen with exclusive breastfeeding. The generalizability of these findings may be limited by participant attrition and by our complete case approach to analysis ....*

They further added:

> *As studies have linked obesity and insulin resistance to difficulties with breastfeeding, suggesting that decreased duration of breastfeeding could be a marker for an existing abnormal metabolic profile, prospective studies are needed to further clarify these relationships. In addition, although we were able to include early adult BMI as a proxy measure of pre-pregnancy adiposity, we were not able to precisely control for pre-gravid abdominal adiposity. We were also limited in our ability to determine whether current visceral fat represented actual gestational weight retained or postpartum weight gained, as a significant period of time had passed between the end of breastfeeding and the assessment of*

adiposity. With a larger sample size, more effects of breastfeeding may have been seen among postmenopausal women. Finally, as breastfeeding may affect adiposity through effects on variables that we entered as covariates in some of our models, it is possible that we have over adjusted some of these models and underestimate the magnitude of the true relationships".

These insightful comments by the authors set out the difficulties of undertaking studies relating breastfeeding to later health, and they provided benchmarks for future studies. These are their key messages:

- gathering prospective data on pre-pregnancy and post-pregnancy health is important
- infant-feeding categories should be compatible with those defined by WHO
- the statistical analysis should be appropriate for addressing all potential confounding factors
- maternal health outcome measures should be assessed *blinded* to infant-feeding data to avoid further bias.

It is also relevant that most of the studies have been undertaken in high-income countries, where durations of breastfeeding are relatively short, and these report positive maternal health effects. For example, consider these four studies:

- Mothers who never breastfed were over five times more likely than those who breastfed all their children for at least three months to have aortic calcification, even after adjustment for socioeconomic status, lifestyle, family history, BMI and traditional risk factors for cardiovascular disease.[5]

- Mothers who breastfed for between seven and twelve months after giving birth for the first time were 28% less likely to develop cardiovascular disease than mothers who never breastfed large US study (called the Women's Health Initiative).[3]

- Mothers who never breastfed, compared to those whose collective lactation period for all their children was two years or more, had a 23% lower risk of coronary heart disease, even after adjustment for age, parity, lifestyle factors, family history and early-adult adiposity.[6]

- Mothers are at a higher risk of type 2 diabetes when full-term pregnancy is followed by up to one month of lactation, independent of physical activity and BMI in later life (thus they should be encouraged to exclusively breastfeed all their infants for at least one month).[4]

Subject to the methodological caveats discussed above, there is evidence that one year of breastfeeding, may provide significant health benefits to the mother. However, the findings of these studies are disparate, and with such disparity it is important to try and disentangle the known and unknown factors that may influence health outcomes. More recently there has been a focus on the *pre-pregnant* health status of mothers, and whether this may influence the decision to breastfeed and therefore explain why women who do not breastfeed have an increased risk of ill-health in later life.[7] Obesity is associated with infertility, spontaneous pregnancy loss and congenital anomalies, and there are metabolic consequences of obesity during pregnancy, whereby obese women have increased insulin resistance in early pregnancy, which manifests in late pregnancy as glucose intolerance and excessive fetal growth. The risk of caesarean section delivery is increased, as are associated wound complications.

After birth, obese women have an increased risk of venous thromboembolism, depression and, importantly, difficulty with breastfeeding. The prevalence of breastfeeding in obese mothers is lower for all categories of breastfeeding, namely 'ever breastfeeding', 'exclusive breastfeeding' and 'continuing breastfeeding'.

In addition, the infants of obese mothers have increased body fat at birth, which may be exacerbated by the early introduction of infant formula and solid foods. Because 50–60% of overweight or obese women gain more weight than recommended during pregnancy, and postpartum weight retention tends to increase, this may lead to increased cardiometabolic risks and other health risks for future pregnancies.

The mechanisms relating adverse perinatal outcomes with maternal obesity are uncertain, but on the basis of the available data it seems that increased pre-pregnancy maternal insulin resistance and accompanying hyperinsulinemia, inflammation and oxidative stress may contribute to early placental and fetal dysfunction.

A recent study on the pre-pregnant health status of mothers reported that poor pre-pregnancy health was associated with reduced prevalence of breastfeeding. When adjustments for the effects of pre-pregnancy health were included in the analysis, the results did not support a causal relationship between longer breastfeeding duration and improved cardiovascular or metabolic health.[7] The authors concluded that it is more likely for pre-pregnant metabolic health to affect both breastfeeding duration and long-term cardiovascular metabolic health. They gave a plausible explanation for the positive findings reported in previous observational studies, namely 'reverse causality', whereby metabolic disease has a negative effect on the prevalence of breastfeeding and evidence of exclusive and continuing breastfeeding is a marker for good pre-pregnancy health status. They further concluded that breastfeeding *per se* does not modify maternal long-term metabolic health.

More findings from the PROBIT study

The PROBIT study examined maternal adiposity outcomes in more than 11,800 mothers at 11.5 years postpartum. The ITT analysis accounted for clustering and provided only weak evidence for any differences in the effects of prolonged breastfeeding compared with control mothers on BMI, fat mass index, fat-free mass index, percentage body fat, and systolic and diastolic blood pressure. The differences were attenuated further when adjustment was made for recruitment of the participants in hospitals or polyclinics, and maternal age, maternal education, smoking habit, and the number of children in the household.[8]

The PROBIT researchers also performed observational analyses, examining the effects of each mother's achieved breastfeeding duration and exclusivity, regardless of whether she was in the breastfeeding promotion group or the control group. This yielded no evidence for an association between 'exclusive breastfeeding' and lower maternal BMI, body fat or systolic blood pressure, or of 'any breastfeeding' with BMI or body fat. There was some indication of lower blood pressure with 'any breastfeeding', although the association was strongest in the group with breastfeeding from six to nine months; and a less strong association with longer durations. 'Exclusive breastfeeding' for six months followed by 'any breastfeeding' for twelve months (as recommended by the American Academy of Pediatrics) was paradoxically associated with somewhat significantly higher maternal BMI and percentage of body fat.

The breastfeeding data of the 'index' (studied) child in each family was combined with infant-feeding data from the mother's subsequent children, to obtain a cumulative duration of lactation for each mother. However, no evidence was found for an effect of cumulative lifetime lactation on any outcome. The study found that in women who initiate breastfeeding, an intervention to promote longer breastfeeding duration did not lead to an important lowering of maternal adiposity or blood pressure.

In conclusion, the current evidence indicates that mothers who have a healthy and normal weight are more likely to choose breastfeeding and to continue breastfeeding for longer than mothers who are overweight/obese and/or have early evidence of metabolic syndrome in the pre-pregnancy period; the latter group of mothers are less likely to breastfeed at all or only breastfeed for a short time, and they are at increased risk of established cardiovascular disease, diabetes mellitus and metabolic syndrome in later life. In this respect, breastfeeding is a marker of pre-pregnancy health.

As mentioned previously, research data on the health benefits of breastfeeding are taken from observational studies because randomized controlled trials of breastfeeding are not possible on ethical grounds. And as explained before, data from observational studies may be influenced by unknown confounding variables. Saying this, pre-pregnancy health status is now being increasingly recognized as a potential factor in later maternal health, and there are likely to be other contributing factors that are as yet unknown.

Breastfeeding and cancer

From a public-health perspective, claims that breastfeeding protects against cancer are a primary focus of investigation. The evidence is predominantly based on observational studies and some case-controlled studies, but no randomized controlled trials.

Breast cancer

Many potential confounding variables including ethnicity, socioeconomic status, diet and lifestyle factors and familial genetic factors relate to breast cancer. Likewise, many confounding factors relate to breastfeeding, many of which overlap with the factors associated with breast cancer. The validity of an outcome therefore depends on the quality and quantity of data available for the known or potentially relevant variables, and how this data is analyzed statistically.

Most breast cancers involve the cells lining the breast ducts. Around 15% of them affect the breast lobules. There are many types and subtypes of breast cancer, classified according to the type of receptor they have (e.g. for oestrogen, progesterone or human epidermal growth factor (hEGF)). Breast cancer cells with or without oestrogen receptors are classified as ER+ or ER−. Those with or without progesterone receptors are PR+ or PR−. And those with hEGF receptors are HER2+ or HER2−. Hormone receptor-positive cancers are the most common subtypes and have a better prognosis than hormone receptor-negative cancers. Note that there may be different effects on risk and prognosis depending on whether the affected woman is pre- or post-menopausal.

Genetic factors are known to play an important role in the development of breast cancer. The term BRCA is an abbreviation for BReast CAncer gene, and *BRCA1* and *BRCA2* are the human genes involved in the production of tumour-suppressor proteins. Everybody has these genes, but mutations of these genes interfere with this process, and without suppressor proteins the risk of someone developing breast cancer increases (as well as other cancers, including ovarian cancer). The mutations are relatively rare, occurring in only one in four hundred people, although the incidence varies according to ethnicity.

The increasing interest in the possible relationship of sub-optimal lactation and later breast cancer has a particular focus on genetic variations that are associated with both conditions.[9-11] The role of genetics as a key modifier of milk production has been recognized for many years in studies undertaken on dairy cattle, but surprisingly little is known about the genes that govern lactation in humans.

Prolactin is the principal lactogenic hormone. It regulates the differentiation of mammary glands and the production of milk. When secreted into the circulation, prolactin binds with receptors known as PRLRs. Prolactin-related genes have been identified in various tissues, including breast, prostate and pancreas, which has led to the evaluation of the effect of prolactin and PRLRs on these tissues, and studies to determine whether genetic expression has a role in the development of cancer. Recent evidence shows that higher levels of prolactin are associated with an increased risk of breast cancer, and a causal relationship between prolactin-receptor expression and breast cancer has been suggested.[12] However, the exact mechanism by which high circulating levels of PRL may influence the risk of cancer is unknown. Several mutations relating to the genetic control of prolactin and prolactin-related (PRLR) genes have been identified in humans and associated with variations in serum prolactin levels.

This emerging area of molecular science needs to be developed further and ultimately translated into the clinical arena. However, it is important for policy-makers and practitioners to be aware that sub-optimal lactation may originate from genetically determined variations in mammary anatomy and physiology. Therefore the advice that every woman is capable of providing sufficient breastmilk for their infant needs to be moderated to reflect the emerging evidence.

From a public-health perspective, there are also several lifestyle factors that may increase the risk of breast cancer. Among them are obesity, smoking habit, alcohol consumption, physical activity, parity, hormone therapy after the menopause, and diabetes mellitus. These factors tend to be more common in women who choose not to breastfeed or who breastfeed for only a short time.

In 2018 the World Cancer Research Fund (WCRF) network reviewed the evidence on the relationship between breastfeeding and cancers of the breast and ovaries. They concluded that breastfeeding *probably* decreases the risk of breast cancer; the evidence for ovarian cancer was *limited but suggestive*.[13] In relation to any dose–response they concluded that *statistically* there was a 2% decrease in the risk of breast cancer per every five months increase in breastfeeding. When pre- and post-menopausal women were considered separately (in a dose–response meta-analysis), the effect of increasing breastfeeding per five-month period was *not* significant, but note that the number of studies in each group was small.[13]

The report of the WCRF included comments about the quality of the data. It was noted that across their studies the measurement of breastfeeding differed –some compared 'ever breastfed' groups with 'never breastfed' groups, thus classifying the duration of breastfeeding was not possible. In other studies, the duration of breastfeeding was self-reported by mothers, which was considered as a potential source of bias. Furthermore, most of the studies were conducted in high-income countries, which generally report shorter durations of breastfeeding than low-income countries, thus (it was commented) the results may not be globally representative

It can be concluded that there needs to be a mechanism for causation, rather than an association, and possible mechanisms may be related to anatomical and physiological changes taking place during lactation, which may offer protection from (or initiate) carcinogenesis. And there may be genetic expressions that relate to the *process* of lactation, that might confer resistance to malignant change. Or it may be that breastfeeding is associated with other lifestyle factors that are known to provide protection against cancer.

Ovarian cancer

Ovarian cancer arises from three different types of cells within the ovary – epithelial cells on the surface of the ovary, stromal cells (that produce oestrogen and progesterone), and germ cells (important in the production of eggs). Some 85–90% of ovarian cancers are epithelial in origin. It has been reported that the risk of developing ovarian cancer is higher in women who have had a higher number of menstrual cycles, which may be associated with not bearing children, having an early menarche, and/or late menopause. A lower risk may be associated with breastfeeding because of the lack of menses during the time of breastfeeding. As with other cancers, several lifestyle factors have been implicated, including oral contraceptives (which may protect against ovarian cancer) and smoking (which may increase the risk), and there may also be familial factors that increase maternal risk. Most ovarian cancers occur spontaneously, but 5–10% relate to genetic predisposition.

The Expert Group advising the WCRF and the American Institute of Cancer Research decided that the evidence for a link between breastfeeding and ovarian cancer was limited, but suggestive.[13] This means that the evidence was inadequate for claiming a probable or convincing causal or protective relationship, but it does suggest a 'direction of effect'. Although the evidence is limited in terms of quantity and quality of data, and sometimes methodologically flawed, it is not possible to make recommendations, and further research on any link between breastfeeding and ovarian cancer is required.

Breastfeeding, cancer and docosahexaenoic acid (DHA)

There has also been increasing interest in the role of the omega-3 long-chain PUFA known as DHA as a factor that may link breastfeeding to breast cancer. Population studies conducted over the last few decades have reported that high levels of fish consumption are related to a lower incidence of breast cancer, suggesting there is a protective role of omega PUFAs. Oily fish is a major dietary source. It has also been noted that rural Japanese people and Eskimos in Greenland, who exhibit low breast cancer rates, consume a larger amount of dietary omega-3 PUFAs than Americans who are at high risk.

Early animal studies have shown that fish oils rich in omega-3 PUFAs, mainly in the form of eicosapentaenoic acid (EPA) and DHA, inhibit tumour development.[14,15] And more recently it has been found that women with evidence of high intake ratios of EPA and DHA, relative to the omega-6 fatty acid arachidonic acid, have a lower risk of breast cancer than those with low ratios of these fats. Interest in the use of omega-3 fatty acid supplements for reducing the risk of cancer and other chronic debilitating conditions (including cardiovascular disease and cognitive impairment) stems from several longstanding lines of investigation. Some of their findings are:

- An increased incidence of breast cancer and heart disease in western societies with low omega-3 to omega-6 fatty acid intake ratios.
- A very low incidence of both of these conditions in populations with high marine omega-3 fatty acid intakes (that is, the Japanese and indigenous Alaskans and Greenlanders).
- A dramatic increase in the incidence of both of these conditions in cohorts from low-incidence populations who migrate to western countries and/or adopt a western diet.

A plausible hypothesis that links dietary DHA, breastfeeding and breast cancer is supported by the following evidence:[14,15]

- The accumulation of DHA in blood and tissues depends on the mother's dietary intake of oily fish.
- The incidence of breast cancer is lowest in countries with a high dietary intake of oily fish.
- DHA is always present in breastmilk and the level relates to the mother's intake of oily fish.
- Mothers with higher dietary fish intake tend to breastfeed for longer.
- DHA has greater anti-inflammatory properties than omega-6 fatty acids (which have pro-inflammatory properties) and the balance between omega-3 and omega-6 influences the risk of inflammatory reactions that may be associated with malignant change.

Most of the research investigating omega-3 fatty acids and cancer has focused on DHA. For example, it is well established that changes in DHA content within the cell membrane have multiple effects in the body, including the modulation of neurological, immune and cardiovascular functions. In breast cancer, for example, DHA increases the sensitivity of breast cancer cells to different chemotherapeutic agents. And in animal models of breast cancer, dietary DHA decreases tumour growth. Preclinical studies have demonstrated that DHA increases the efficacy of both doxorubicin and docetaxel, two agents commonly used as 'adjuvants' for breast-cancer treatment. Increased levels of DHA in breast adipose tissue have been found to correlate with a *better* response to chemotherapy. And an increased dietary intake of omega-3 long chain PUFA, including DHA, results in increased incorporation of DHA into breast adipose tissue.

A recent meta-analysis combined six prospective case–control studies and five cohort studies in which the omega-3 to omega-6 dietary intake ratios were known, as well as the omega-3 to omega-6 ratios of their phospholipid forms in serum.[15] There were a total of more than 274,000 women in these studies, and more than 8,300 breast cancer events. The authors' conclusions were that each 1 in 10 increments in the dietary ratio of omega-3 to omega-6 was associated with a 6% reduction in the risk of breast cancer. Among the US participants, each one in ten increment in the serum ratio of omega-3 to omega-6 phospholipids was associated with a 27% reduction in breast cancer risk.

Compelling though this evidence is, bear in mind that this is all work in progress (like the genetic studies described above). The information gleaned has been highlighted here to underline the importance of research findings that may modify the information we currently provide to parents about breastfeeding and cancer. As it is the most common cancer in women, high-quality research must continue, with a focus on *causal* mechanisms and establishing the best treatment.

Conclusion

It is clearly important that any information about the health benefits of breastfeeding is an accurate reflection of the available evidence, and that it is presented to parents in a form that not only sets out the potential benefits but also clarifies any potential weaknesses in the evidence. In preparing manuscripts for submission to scientific journals, authors are encouraged to note the strengths and weaknesses or limitations of their work, as done by the authors of some of the papers referred to in this chapter, who acknowledge that further studies are required. The problem is that these caveats relating to results and data tend not to be included in the information subsequently provided to parents through WHO, activists, industry and media outlets. Unlike health claims for nutrients and nutritional products, there is no regulatory process for the promotion and marketing of breastfeeding, so it is important that an eagerness to support breastfeeding does not lead to claims of health benefits that are not in keeping with the available scientific evidence.

A key issue lies in the way 'associations' between breastfeeding and the ever-increasing number of health conditions are interpreted. It is important to acknowledge that any information on health and breastfeeding should be accompanied by a level (of certainty or uncertainty) for each association or health claim.

As discussed earlier, this could be one of the functions of an independent Global Research Advisory Centre. It could be affiliated with a relevant academic centre of excellence. It could provide advice to researchers and policy-makers on the priorities for investigating infant and young-child feeding, and share the learning from previous studies, highlighting the critical elements of study design and methodology. It could also act as a data-monitoring and coordinating centre and ensure that content and dissemination of research information is appropriate for the level of certainty of the scientific evidence. With a major source of the underlying stakeholder conflict being the variation in interpretation of the available research data, an independent advisory input may bring a more balanced and reliable approach to the policy-making process.

References

1. Louis-Jacques A, Stuebe A (2018) Long-term maternal benefits of breastfeeding. *Contemporary Obstetrics and Gynecology Journal* 64(7), 26–29. Available at: https://www.contemporaryobgyn.net/view/long-term-maternal-benefits-breastfeeding (last accessed August 2022).

2. McNeilly A (1969) Breastfeeding and the suppression of fertility. *Food and Nutrition Bulletin* 17, 163.

3. Schwarz EB, Ray RM, Stuebe AM, *et al.* (2009) Duration of lactation and risk factors for maternal cardiovascular disease. *Obstetrics and Gynecology* 113, 974–82. Available at: https://www.ncbi.nlm.nih.gov/pmc/articles/PMC2714700/ (last accessed August 2022).

4. Schwarz EB, Brown JS, Creasman JM, *et al.* (2010) Lactation and maternal risk of type 2 diabetes: a population-based study. *American Journal of Medicine* 123, 863, e1–6. Available at: https://www.amjmed.com/article/S0002-934310)00385-2/fulltext (last accessed August 2022).

5. Schwarz EB, McClure CK, Tepper PG, *et al.* (2010) Lactation and maternal measures of subclinical cardiovascular disease. *Obstetrics and Gynecology* 115(1), 41–48.

6. Stuebe AM, Michels KB, Willett WC, *et al.* (2009) Duration of lactation and incidence of myocardial infarction in middle to late adulthood. *American Journal of Obstetrics and Gynecology* 138, e1–e8.

7. Velle-Forbord V, Skrastad RB, Salvesen O, *et al.* (2019) Breastfeeding and long-term maternal metabolic health in the HUNT study: a longitudinal population-based cohort study. *British Journal of Obstetrics and Gynaecology* 126, 526–34.

8. Oken E, Patel R, Guthrie LB, *et al.* (2013) Effects of an intervention to promote breastfeeding on maternal adiposity and blood pressure at 11.5 years postpartum: results from the Promotion of Breastfeeding Intervention Trial, a cluster-randomized controlled trial. *American Journal of Clinical Nutrition* 98, 1048–56. Available at: https://pubmed.ncbi.nlm.nih.gov/23945719/ (last accessed August 2022).

9. Lee S, Kelleher SL (2016) Biological underpinnings of breastfeeding challenges: the role of genetics, diet, and environment on lactation physiology. *American Journal of Physiology Endocrinology and Metabolism* 311, E405–22. DOI:10.1152/ajpendo.00495.2015.

10. Kelleher SL, Gagnon A, Riveraet OC, *et al.* (2019) Milk-derived miRNA profiles elucidate molecular pathways that underlie breast dysfunction in women with common genetic variants in *SLC30A2*. *Sci Rep* **9,** 12686 Available at: https://www.ncbi.nlm.nih.gov/pmc/articles/PMC6722070/ (last accessed August 2022).

11. Sethi BK, Chanukya GV, Nagesh VS (2016) Prolactin and cancer: has the orphan finally found a home? *Indian Journal of Endocrinology and Metabolism* 16(Suppl. S2), 195–98.

12. Golan Y, Assaraf YG (2020) Genetic and physiological factors affecting human milk production and composition. *Nutrients* 12, 1500.

13. World Cancer Research Fund/American Institute for Cancer Research. Continuous Update Project Expert Report (2018) *Lactation and the risk of cancer*. Available at: https://www.wcrf.org/wp-content/uploads/2021/02/Lactation.pdf (last accessed August 2022).

14. Fabian CJ, Kimler BF, Hursting SD (2015) Omega-3 fatty acids for breast cancer prevention and survivorship. *Breast Cancer Research* 17, 62. Available at: https://breast-cancer-research.biomedcentral.com/articles/10.1186/s13058-015-0571-6 (last accessed August 2022).

15. Yang B, Ren XL, Fu YQ, *et al.* (2014) Ratio of *n-3*/*n-6* PUFAs and risk of breast cancer: a meta-analysis of 274135 adult females from 11 independent prospective studies. *BMC Cancer* 14, 105.

CHAPTER 12

Interest groups, advocates and activists

Interest groups are a key element of modern society and in healthcare it can be argued that the quality of a healthcare system depends not only on the best science and clinical practice, but also on the extent to which health organizations are willing to engage with civil society and – in particular – with special interest groups.

A plethora of groups have focused on infant and young-child feeding, almost entirely with a special interest in breastfeeding. The nature and structure of these interest groups varies from single small groups, such as community breastfeeding support groups, to international campaigning organizations such as IBFAN. Some of them merge to form coalitions, such as the Global Breastfeeding Collective initiative which is a partnership of at least twenty-five global breastfeeding organizations and is led by UNICEF and WHO.[1]

The profile of these organizations differs from providing support to local breastfeeding mothers, to undertaking international campaigns against global infant-formula companies. In the 1970s and 80s the campaigning groups were highly successful in raising awareness of the consequences of commercial marketing of infant formulas in the most deprived parts of the world. This action subsequently led to WHO publishing the Code.

Special interest, advocates and activists

Across the spectrum of civil interest in infant and child feeding there are varying degrees of activism. Special interest and advocacy groups generally contribute to and collaborate within national and local health systems, whereas activists tend to spread their protests and actions across a range of related organizations – both national and international – to achieve their core objectives.

This is the pattern in relation to breastfeeding, with support and advocacy focusing on the healthcare system. But campaigning activists, such as IBFAN, target WHO, governments, the media and academia, as well as industry and healthcare. It is interesting that activism in infant and young-child feeding is almost entirely focused on breastfeeding. Although this has undoubtedly highlighted the importance of breastfeeding, there is some concern that it has also detracted from the other key elements of infant and young-child nutrition.

In developing countries, the inadequacy of maternal nutrition, failure to provide nutritious complementary foods and deficiencies in family diets are equally important if the health and wellbeing of infants and young children are to be optimized. In developed countries, widespread child obesity predisposes to a range of chronic adult diseases that shorten life expectancy. More recently, attention has been drawn to the double burden of malnutrition, which is increasingly prevalent in countries with emerging economies and relates to children who are not only overweight or obese but also malnourished.[2]

It is not clear why there is such a dominant emphasis on one specific aspect of the infant and young child diet at the expense of others – and why there is not a holistic approach for all aspects of diet, from birth to three years and beyond, to ensure that children's nutritional requirements during this important period of rapid growth and development are being met.[3]

Simultaneously up-scaling both breastfeeding and complementary feeding would surely be the most sensible way forward, and this should be central to strategic planning. However, WHO continues to see breastfeeding and complementary feeding as separate entities, as noted in the establishment of the Global Breastfeeding Collective. This raises two questions:

- Why is this not an infant and young-child feeding collective with special interest, advocate and activist groups also focusing on complementary feeding?
- Why is complementary feeding neglected, when from the age of six months it plays such a critical role in determining normal growth and development during early life and beyond?

With WHO's preferred allegiance being with breastfeeding activist groups, should this be considered as a material conflict of interest? And is a declaration required when consideration is being given (or not being given) to matters that relate to other aspects of infant feeding and practice? Otherwise, can the majority of parents – who are not activists – have confidence that WHO's relationship with breastfeeding activist organizations will not prejudice the importance of avoiding systematic bias within the policy-making process.

The Global Breastfeeding Collective

On 1 August 2017, the Global Breastfeeding Collective was presented as a partnership of international agencies including WHO and UNICEF, who are calling on donors, policymakers, philanthropists and civil society to increase investment in breastfeeding worldwide.[1] The Collective's vision is of a world in which all mothers have the financial, emotional, technical and public support they need to start breastfeeding within an hour of a child's birth, then to breastfeed exclusively for six months, and to continue breastfeeding (with adequate, age-appropriate and safe complementary foods) for two years or beyond. The Collective advocates for 'smart investments' in breastfeeding, to help policymakers and NGOs implement solutions and galvanize public support and thus get real results in terms of increased rates of breastfeeding for children, families and nations. The Collective has four strategic goals:

- to foster leadership and alliances to galvanize support to breastfeeding
- to effectively integrate and communicate breastfeeding messages to reach strategic audiences
- to mobilize resources and promote accountability, and
- to build knowledge and evidence to enhance breastfeeding policies, programmes, financing and communication.

As previously indicated, what is most remarkable about this initiative is that although reference may be made to other aspects of infant and young-child feeding that are also fundamentally important, there is not the same commitment. Breastfeeding may be the sole nutrition during the first six months of life, but thereafter it is just one component of a feeding programme, whereby each food entity should complement the others and thus provide a diet that meets the infant or young child's requirements at the time.

Membership of the Global Breastfeeding Collective is clearly the 'hot ticket' for breastfeeding activists, and applicants are required to demonstrate a significant contribution to the protection, promotion and support of breastfeeding (which may include technical or financial assistance to breastfeeding programmes), in addition to demonstrating willingness to contribute to the advancement of the strategic goals of the Collective. UNICEF and WHO review the declaration of interest of potential members and decide on membership in line with UNICEF and WHO policies and rules. There is a Coordination Committee that includes permanent representation from UNICEF and WHO and six other members are elected. The Coordination Committee functions as the decision-making body.

It is unfortunate that the terms of reference for membership of the Collective make no reference to the other critically important nutritive and non-nutritive factors that influence the nutritional status of infants and young children. The Collective is clearly a group of like-minded organizations and individuals, carefully selected on the basis of their breastfeeding credentials by WHO and UNICEF, but this may raise concerns of segregation within the wider infant-feeding community. With the high levels of chumocracy and this 'closed shop' approach, it may be presumed that the views and proposals of the Collective will be fast-tracked through the WHO and UNICEF decision-making systems, thereby avoiding wider consultation. It is difficult not to conclude that there is a high risk of conflict of interest within this structure, thus the governance arrangements need to be transparent and should cover issues such as moral, ethical, professional and financial standards. For this to be achieved and provide appropriate assurances, the process needs to be independently regulated.

At the time of the launch of the Collective, the UNICEF Executive Director was quoted as saying:

> *"What if governments had a proven, cost-effective way to save babies' lives, reduce rates of malnutrition, support children's health, increase educational attainment and grow productivity? They do: it's called breastfeeding. And it is one of the best investments nations can make in the lives and futures of their youngest members – and in the long-term strength of their societies".*

To some extent this may be true, but these words would be more appropriate and convincing if they were applied to the benefits of a nutritionally balanced diet throughout childhood. If the diet is optimal, and a child receives foods that bring a balanced diversity to their diet, it can be anticipated that the magnitude of benefit from preventing malnutrition, wasting, stunting, obesity and other causes of early life morbidity and mortality, will greatly exceed the potential benefits that are limited to breastmilk – even if the mother and child fulfil the breastfeeding recommendations of the WHO policy.

The role of WHO and UNICEF is surprising, and it raises questions about whether their global infant feeding responsibilities are being influenced by their obvious preference towards breastfeeding and their antipathy towards the infant-food industry This may be negatively impacting on the wider nutritional and healthcare needs of infants and children worldwide. It is evident from the mission of the Collective that achieving an integrated approach to *all* aspects of infant feeding is not an objective that the Collective and their members have identified as a priority. On the one hand there is the Collective's message of breastfeeding supremacy; and on the other there is the segregation and discrimination of infants and their families who (for justifiable reasons) are not breastfeeding activists, who will not commit to this type of propaganda and self-interest. With WHO and UNICEF placing themselves at the extreme end of the infant-feeding policy spectrum, a social consensus with a meeting of minds between ideologists and realists remains unlikely.

It is therefore important for organizations that have committed to support the Collective on breastfeeding matters to appreciate the wider needs of infant and child nutrition and their related health, and recognize the dangers and limitations of infant-feeding policy only being seen through the prism of breastfeeding. They need to appreciate that the potential health benefits of breastfeeding are diminished by collateral factors such as:

- malnutrition of both mother and child
- the lack of local produce and failure to have appropriate food-supply chains
- non-nutritive issues such as contaminated water, poor sanitation and poor housing
- the lack of safe cooking facilities, and
- living with inadequate healthcare and education provision.

WHO and activism

The close relationship between WHO and breastfeeding activist groups is based on a shared view of how they see breastfeeding policy developing currently, and presumably in the future. The problem is that their vision is highly ideological. Stakeholders who are more closely involved at a grass-roots level, particularly health professionals and parents, believe that change should be realistic and incremental. Although it would be wonderful to envisage an infant-feeding utopia, whereby all women worldwide breastfeed for two years or beyond, have access to a plentiful supply of nutritious complementary foods, use no infant formula, have adequate resources for research and education, enjoy improved social circumstances with suitable housing that has a clean water supply and decent sanitation, and receive a household income that meets all the family's needs. However, the truth is, this will never be achieved by *all* families, and therefore policy needs to reflect the reality. This is why it is so important for ideologists and realists to work together to determine the greatest need, and to prioritize the actions that are required.

And this needs to be conducted in a spirit of common understanding, in which the value of compromise is recognized, and there is engagement with all key stakeholders– especially parents.

The increasingly close bond between WHO and interest groups was evident with the establishment of NetCode, a system that monitors compliance with the Code.[4] Having established this new system, their stated objective is to:

> *"... hold manufacturers, distributors, retail outlets, the healthcare system and healthcare workers to account for their breaches of national laws and/or the Code".[4]*

There is, however, a significant conflict of interest because WHO and other breastfeeding activist groups are in effect acting as lawmaker, prosecutor, judge, jury and executioner. This is unusual, as judicial processes should be independent of lawmakers and prosecution services. The distinction between a prosecutor in charge of an investigation and a judge in charge of adjudication is at the basis of most criminal justice systems. Ensuring judges are not directly involved in the processes of investigation and prosecution safeguards the neutral and detached position of the judicial process. The role of a judge is to apply the law – not be involved in setting the law – therefore there is a clear separation between judges and lawmakers.

There are therefore several aspects of NetCode that do not comply with these principles, including WHO and breastfeeding activists who are setting the rules and then adjudicating on alleged non-compliance. The overarching impression is that the system appears to allow the least-regulated infant-feeding organizations to regulate the most-regulated organizations, rather than vice versa. In relation to previous comments on the role of sponsorship, NetCode has been sponsored by the Bill & Melinda Gates Foundation. Whether this is an acceptable arrangement is difficult to determine without details of the engagement or declarations of interest and any associated governance standards.

As with all conflicts the various parties tend to blame each other and this is apparent in the process of setting infant-feeding policy. This is despite a clear message from behaviour scientists that if you want to motivate behavioural change, do not engage in the 'blame game' because it is ineffective and damaging.[5] In relation to policy-making, it is a retrograde step to ascribe blame and assert culpability without allowing for the evaluation of the character and value of a policy to be fully accepted. What is particularly frustrating to some is that the general substance of infant-feeding policy is welcomed by all stakeholders, and the source of the blame behaviour predominantly relates to small, although significant, details, such as the timings for exclusive breastfeeding and introduction of complementary feeding, and the duration of continuing breastfeeding. The transitions in diet are understood, but there is reticence about the specific timings which, at the extremes, are considered by some to be excessively aspirational rather that evidential.

Instead of collectively re-visiting these contentious details, the trend has been for a hardening of views by WHO and activist groups, accompanied by a desire to resort to legislation. This approach contrasts with the view that policy-making needs to motivate behaviour change. For this to be achieved decisions must be made within the spirit of acknowledging credit and avoiding blame.

Further evidence that WHO and activist relationship may need closer governance and surveillance was evident in relation to the issue of inappropriate marketing and promotion of breastmilk substitutes, which included WHO's re-interpretation of the term 'breastmilk substitutes'.[6] Following the WHA meeting in 2016, at which the issue was considered, Baby Milk Action posted a photograph on their website showing WHO officials and IBFAN members celebrating the outcome of WHA resolution 69.9 (see www.babymilkaction.org/archives/9771) (this is also discussed on page 106). However, subsequent events may portray this as a pyrrhic victory. The photograph gave the impression that resolution WHA 69.9 and the guidance prepared by WHO Secretariat were both adopted at the 2016 WHA, but at a subsequent meeting of the Codex Committee on Nutrition and Foods for Special Dietary Uses, the assumed adoption of the guidance was questioned by the French delegation. This precipitated a response from a WHO representative (who featured in the photograph) that the documentation was *"welcomed with appreciation"* and in WHO language this has the same meaning as 'adopted, approved and endorsed', and therefore indicating that both the resolution and the guidance *were* adopted.

This deduction was subsequently corrected by WHO's Office of the Legal Counsel, which emphasized the following:

> *"… it should be noted that the Guidance was not approved or endorsed but was welcomed with appreciation. … Welcomed with appreciation is not synonymous with approved".*

An extract from the notification from the WHO's Office of the Legal Counsel is shown in Box 12.1 *overpage*. It is not surprising that suspicions have been raised over the role of WHO and their relationship with activist groups on this matter,

Box 12.1: Extract from the Joint FAO/WHO Standards Programme Codex Committee on Nutrition and Foods for Special Dietary Uses (39th session, Berlin, Germany, 4–8 December 2017)

I. Matters or interest arising from FAO and WHO
CX/NFSDU 17/39/3 Addendum 14
Addendum: Correction by the WHO office of the Legal Counsel

Whereas it is stated on page 6 of the document that the WHO Technical Guidance on Ending the Inappropriate Promotion of Foods for Infants and Young Children was approved by the 69th WHA through resolution WHA 69.9, it should be noted that this Guidance was not approved or endorsed, but was welcomed with appreciation (see operative paragraph 1 of resolution WHA 69.9).

Resolution WHA 69.9 itself (i.e. the resolution as a whole) was adopted by consensus on 28 May 2016 at the eighth plenary meeting of the 69th WHA.

It is WHO member states that give meaning to the language they use.

Furthermore, in WHO practice, operative terms such as "welcomes", "welcomes with appreciation", "notes" and "notes with appreciation" have different meanings and are not use synonymously with the term "approves".

and whether the outcome is a reflection of collaboration or collusion. The photograph taken post-resolution of WHO officials, IBFAN representatives and the Chair of the Working Group (Fig 7.1) may influence your opinion.

With the WHA being the decision-making body, and decisions are being considered by government representatives from 194 countries, it is inevitable that there will situations where agreement on wording of resolutions can be a tortuous process and this was apparently evident during the formulation of the final version of resolution 69.9 in the days immediately before its agreement at WHA.

A patchwork of politics and self-interest (involving a hundred and ninety-four countries and their official representatives, and several observer groups, including well-prepared activist organizations) may not reflect the expectations of parents who will understandably be expecting WHO to be carefully addressing the nutritional interests of their children; and that policy will be based on obtaining the best scientific evidence and advice from the most informed researchers and clinicians worldwide.

The reality, it seems to be, is that the WHA decision-making process is highly political and influenced by competing interests, and it will continue to be blighted by conflict, division and political turmoil as long as there is a lack of robust governance systems.

Effective governance structures will acknowledge that special interest and activist groups *do* have a role to play in raising standards and ensuring that parents are adequately supported in all aspects of infant and young-child feeding. However, it should also be recognized that all stakeholders need to have a clear understanding of their function within the multidisciplinary approach to infant feeding.

Activists do not have day-to-day responsibility for the delivery of child health services, so while their focus on breastfeeding is important it may also need to be compatible with the wider aspects of the delivery of services for infant and young-child feeding.

This point highlights the difficulty of aligning ideological preferences with the need to face real-world circumstances. And this is why WHO's leadership of infant and young-child nutrition should take a broader view – to ensure that the policy approach is comprehensive and deliverable and does not create harm by neglecting key elements of other aspects of nutritional care.

WHO has a responsibility for ensuring that the infant and young-child diet will address nutritional requirements for *all* children during early life, and the challenges of meeting this objective will extend well beyond breastfeeding.

How could this be managed differently?

Each stakeholder has a different professional background, and it is important that they are all allowed to contribute and deliver their views, from their own perspective. Their presence and contributions should be subject to agreed professional, governance and regulatory standards. The WHO needs to demonstrate that it is a leader to *all* stakeholders and that it is able to exhibit the professional standards that are expected of an international leader in such an important aspect of global health.

Effective leadership requires vision, strategic thinking and focus, but also integrity, cooperation and humility. It is the latter attribute that will facilitate engagement, support and respect. Campaigners must influence and deliver their message but should at the same time adopt professional standards for partnership-working.

Would a more moderate approach to activism in the area of infant and young-child feeding be more effective? Although the context and narrative may be similar, the difference between extremism and moderation is that the boundaries are in different places. This concept would certainly apply to the controversy surrounding infant-feeding policy whereby the boundaries applied by WHO and breastfeeding activist groups are not compliant with that of the general population. In these circumstances, moderation would involve greater sensitivity to the needs and wishes of parents, greater flexibility in determining infant-feeding goals, and greater understanding of the collateral factors that influence future choices and decisions. It is not surprising that within the breastfeeding interest groups there are varying degrees of extremism and moderation, as was noted in 2013 in the Save the Children Fund document entitled *Superfood for Babies*. This document opened the door for industry to participate in policy discussions, but the opportunity has not been taken by other campaigners (see Box 12.2).

Box 12.2: Industry involvement in policy-activist views

Statement in the International Code (1981)

Affirming the need for governments, organisations, or the United Nations system, non-governmental organisations, experts in various related disciplines, consumer groups and industry to cooperate in activities aimed at the improvement of maternal, infant, and young child health and Nutrition.

Statement in the *Superfood for Babies* (Save the Children, 2013)

While we acknowledge that the industry has a valuable role to play in policymaking, it should be as transparent as possible to ensure there is no undue influence on governments and legislative processes."

Health professionals have to take a more proactive approach to infant feeding and policy to ensure that policy decisions do not conflict with best practice for individual children. Health professionals are not usually reticent when it comes to expressing their views on health matters and it is therefore interesting that very few openly challenge issues about infant feeding – especially if they are in conflict with WHO's recommendations – nor do they tend to question specific evidence in relation to breastfeeding. It is evident from informal murmurings that their silence may not reflect their accordance, and individuals and organizations are choosing to avoid potential opposition from WHO and breastfeeding-support organizations, thus they choose to focus their knowledge and expertise on other health issues. However, health professionals do need to contribute, and to share their views, and give their support to a vulnerable population within society that cannot represent itself. It is obviously important to have open discussions that allow an exchange of ideas, and these are conducted in a respectful and professional manner. There are too many historical examples of the health and welfare of children suffering as a consequence of institutional authoritarianism suppressing voices of concern.

It goes without saying that parents need to be more closely involved with each of the stakeholders if they are going to be in a position to understand the issues, and make the best decisions for their children. The power of people working together cannot not be underestimated. A collective ethos behind a project as important as infant and young-child policy-making is the key to achieving the overall goal of attaining the best health and wellbeing for all children. In stark contrast, dysfunctional behaviours are destructive and intolerable, and they cost lives.

References

1. WHO/UNICEF (2017) *Global Breastfeeding Collective*. Available at: https://www.globalbreastfeedingcollective.org/ (last accessed August 2022).

2. Branca F, Demaio A, Udomkesmalee E, *et al.* (2020) A new nutrition manifesto for a new nutrition reality. *The Lancet* 395, 8–10.

3. Victora CG, Bahl R, Barros AJD, *et al.* (2016) Breastfeeding in the 21st century: epidemiology, mechanisms, and lifelong effect. *The Lancet* 38, 475–90.

4. WHO/UN Children's Fund (2017) *NetCode toolkit. Monitoring the marketing of breastmilk substitutes: protocol for ongoing monitoring systems*. Licence CC BY-NC-SA 3.0 IGO. Available at: https://apps.who.int/iris/bitstream/handle/10665/259441/9789241513180-eng.pdf?sequence=1&isAllowed=y (last accessed August 2022).

5. Leong C, Howlett M (2017) On credit and blame: disentangling the motivations of public policy decision-making behaviour. *Policy Science* 50, 599–618. Available at: https://link.springer.com/article/10.1007/s11077-017-9290-4 (last accessed August 2022?).

6. *WHO (2016) Maternal, infant, and young child nutrition. Guidance on Ending the Inappropriate Promotion of Foods for Infants and Young Children. 69th WHA Document A69/7 Add.1 2016*. Available at: http://apps.who.int/gb/ebwha/pdf_files/WHA69/A69_7Add1-en.pdf?ua=1&ua=1/ (last accessed August 2022).

CHAPTER 13

Dysfunctional partnership-working

In the recent *Lancet* series on the double burden of malnutrition[1] it is acknowledged that effective partnership-working is essential. The named stakeholder groups are governments, the UN, civil society, academia, media, philanthropy and multi-bilaterals, private sector and regional economic platforms. *The Lancet* paper to which I refer is entitled 'A new nutrition manifesto for a new nutrition reality' and the lead author is the Director of the Department of Nutrition for Health and Development at WHO. The article clearly states that the authors have no intention of resolving the longstanding conflict between WHO and the infant-food industry and, in so doing, expect the other stakeholders to accede to more decades of acrimony and division. They state that:

> "*Although new strategic partnerships are essential, we must recognize the damage and mistrust that result from incompatible partnerships with stakeholders whose behaviour runs counter to human or planetary health. The food industry has an important role in implementing and delivering change. However, companies cannot be allowed to influence and interfere in public policy making or bias the science that underpins this process. While constructive dialogue is necessary, a default seat at the table for private-sector representatives should not be assumed and policy development processes need to be firewalled from vested interests*".[1]

Do the authors believe that these comments only apply to industry? Do they really expect that the wider infant-feeding community, including health professionals and parents, believe that all of the other representatives do not have a vested interest, including WHO, or will not attempt to influence public policy-making or challenge the science? It could be argued that if they are not doing that, why are they there?

Moreover, what right do these authors have to make this decision? Must we remind ourselves that the key products for the provision of nutrition and health care in early life are breastmilk, infant formula as a safety net, and complementary foods, with the stakeholders responsible for delivering these products to infants being parents, health professionals, and the infant food industry, none of whom are mentioned in the long list of 'named stakeholders'?

By turning their backs on the infant-formula industry, these stakeholders are turning their backs on infants who require a safe alternative to breastmilk. Many of these infants will already be disadvantaged when they enter this world. Why do policy-makers and eminent scientists wish to create even greater inequality?

The exclusion of industry over many years has not enabled breastfeeding targets to be met, it has not ensured that infants worldwide receive nutritionally adequate complementary foods, and it has not prevented the rapidly emerging double burden of malnutrition.

An independent review would want to determine whether the absence of industry at the policy-making table has mitigated or compounded these disappointing outcome measures. Similarly, they will want to assess the performance of the organizations who were given the responsibility for protecting infants and young children from substandard nutrition.

The statement in *The Lancet* suggests that the food industry should be held responsible for deteriorating planetary health, which is a new assertion, which surprisingly comes from the organization that, since 1948, has been responsible for directing and coordinating international health.

WHO and industry

It is remarkable that with this background, of failure to provide the right food to the right children, it is not thought necessary to have individuals from the food industry who are experts in food science, food manufacture, food distribution and food safety, who can make valuable contributions to the stakeholder discussions. If it is intended to include a wider range of stakeholders, it is important that these advocates for planetary health, faith-based leaders, innovators and investors have the opportunity to meet and discuss the issues with experts from the food industry and thus allow all stakeholders to develop their own thoughts and conclusions about whether industry should contribute to the planning and delivery of the best nutrition for infants and children worldwide.

They may feel that rather than continue with an arrangement that has failed to bring about change, industry involvement, supported by robust peer governance, may be a more effective way forward. They may also find that there are some important developments upon which working relations can build, such as the Nestlé global climate roadmap to halve greenhouse-gas emissions by 2030 and reach net zero by 2050 (see: https://www.nestle.co.uk/en-gb/sustainability/climate-change.

As the old nutrition ideology is not working, a 'new nutrition reality' requires new thinking and new people. Simply wiping the slate clean and starting again with the same preferences and prejudices is not acceptable. Among the new stakeholders, industry should be represented by colleagues who will bring an aspect of science and technology that will not be widely available from the other stakeholder representatives. Moreover, it will be the quality of the leadership that will determine whether industry can change from being the *bête noire* of infant feeding to becoming a valued partner in the planning and development of infant and young-child nutrition.

There appears to be an assumption that scientists undertaking nutrition research in industry are less trustworthy than those working in an academic environment. This inference is not accompanied by material evidence, so this thinking has to be strongly challenged. Scientists and clinicians working in both academia *and* industry have the potential to provide the foundation for exciting new developments in all aspects of nutrition and healthcare; their contribution should therefore be commended, rather than denigrated, by WHO officials. It is critically important that scientists are able to collaborate to produce the best evidence regarding the optimum nutrition for infants and children worldwide. During the coronavirus pandemic, WHO, governments, industry and scientists from academia and industry have worked together to develop diagnostic tests, treatments and vaccines and their contribution to controlling this infection has been lauded.

The longstanding heavy mortality of children under five years of age from nutrition-related causes is not only a consequence of the low priority this issue has been given by governments, but is also a failure of policy-makers to underline the importance of encouraging all academics (those in industry and those in universities) to focus on developing nutritional solutions to the childhood nutritional pandemic. It is surprising that the authors of this *Lancet* article, many of whom are eminent academics, should be content to exile fellow scientists who are undertaking original research in world-class research laboratories, on the grounds that they are working in an industry environment. Research misconduct can occur in all institutions, including the most eminent academic centres, and at all levels, including the individual researcher, the department, the institution, the scientific journals, and the funding bodies. Bias in educational articles can reflect many factors, including associations with research funding organizations, government bodies, industry, or simply being employed by a university with a policy of 'publish or perish'. Discrimination against academics employed by industry is a dangerous precedent.

Depending upon the agenda, it would make sense to consider whether the contribution from the scientific or the business element of industry is appropriate. The current practice of excluding the whole of industry because of issues relating to marketing and sales of products has not worked and the positions of WHO and industry have in the meantime become more entrenched. Having a relationship on the scientific aspects of infant formulas and foods may create a more constructive environment and allow progress to be made on non-compliance with the Code.

Intelligent and capable leadership should be able to separate the industry contribution to academia from the industry contribution to business and both of these aspects of industry need separate solutions. From an industry perspective, the marketing and sales departments should not be allowed to make statements that misinterpret evidence from scientific research undertaken within academia, and WHO and other policy-makers should not discriminate against good-quality research simply because it was undertaken in an industry environment.

The current stance on this issue lacks intellectual finesse and is impacting negatively on the wider issues of research and development. For example, to undertake clinical intervention studies the quality and safety standards of the intervention product need to be of the highest level with technological expertise that is not available even in the most prestigious university research units. Collaborative research should be covered by a shared governance approach and thus allow industry and university scientists, and their respective clinicians, to work together without fear of unsubstantiated claims of conflict of interest.

Industry and governance

There is a precedent of industry collaborating with academia and the public sector. The International Life Sciences Institute (ILSI) was founded in 1978 as a non-profit, worldwide organization whose mission is to provide science that improves human health and wellbeing and safeguards the environment.[2] The European Branch of ILSI (ILSI Europe) was created in 1986 and fosters collaboration among the best scientists from industry, academia and the public sector to provide evidence-based scientific solutions that pave the way to enhanced nutrition, food safety, consumer trust and sustainability. To deliver science of the highest quality and integrity, the scientists collaborate and share their expertise in expert groups, workshops, symposia and publications.

ILSI Europe is funded primarily by its industry members, and other sources including the European Commission when participating as a partner in EU-funded projects. There are robust governance systems underpinning these arrangements. The EU has renewed ILSI Europe's transparency status, confirming that ILSI Europe continues to comply with the EU Transparency Register, which is located under the NGOs section of the registry. Important developments in nutrition and food are addressed by the expert groups and the outputs from these activities are published in high-quality scientific journals. The authors of these articles, with researchers from across the academic and industry environment, highlights the evidence of effective collaboration.

In relation to governance it is important to acknowledge that the major infant formula companies have responded to criticism regarding non-compliance and their irresponsible marketing and sales activities, and they are taking measures to improve performance and governance standards.[14] Both Nestlé and Danone have been assessed by FTSE4Good, which is a responsible investment index designed to help investors identify companies that meet globally recognized corporate responsibility standards and it is the only investment index that has defined objective criteria on the responsible marketing of breastmilk substitutes.[3] Nestlé was successful in being added to the index in 2011 and Danone was added in 2016 (for more detail, see Chapter 14). The Access to Nutrition Foundation rates food and beverage manufacturers on their nutrition-related policies, practices, and performance through the two-yearly publication of the global *Access to Nutrition Index*. In 2016, six manufacturers of infant formulas were assessed, and Nestlé and Danone were the highest ranked companies.[4] Both assessments refer to the Code and subsequent resolutions, and to information that is gathered at selected country visits; the assessments continue to evolve in response to comments and criticisms. Not surprisingly WHO and their colleagues in breastfeeding support groups are critical of these initiatives, however they do provide a degree of independence which is not apparent in NetCode, a monitoring system established by WHO[5] (Chapter 14).

If industry is included as an active member of a stakeholder partnership addressing issues of infant feeding, it would offer an opportunity for other partners to observe industry from a governance perspective. Informally, NGOs that are involved in relief work and community development have stated that they see benefits of their organization working with industry, including infant-food companies, because this can provide sustainability for their community projects, by increasing opportunities to create jobs, income and community investment. Moreover, they have emphasized that partnership-working is an effective way of monitoring governance standards of other partners.

With the long history of conflict, it is understandable that some will be wary of direct involvement of industry, and there are others who will firmly resist the suggestion. The strongest argument for calling for change is that forty years is more than enough time for testing the effect of exclusion of industry from partnership-working. And as this has proved to be unsuccessful, new thinking is required.

Infant formula undoubtedly saves lives if breastmilk is not available, and the Code makes reference to the importance of the availability of infant formula. Deliberations on infant formula and the role of industry should therefore reflect on the need for an infant-formula safety net, and the assurance that this provides for parents and also for stakeholders, which should be considered as sufficient justification for industry to contribute to stakeholder discussion.

Any invitation to industry to become an accepted stakeholder will have to be accompanied by conditions that ensure commitment to agreed policies and standards, good governance and regulation, and trust and respect. This could be consolidated in a memorandum of understanding or a similar form of agreement (see Chapter 17). It is therefore proposed that WHO should relax its policy of non-cooperation with industry. It is morally wrong for the organization with global responsibility for infant and young-child feeding to *not* have a professional working relationship with the largest food and beverage company worldwide. Collateral damage is impacting on all stakeholders, including health practitioners and families who clearly support the need for a nutritional safety net for infants who do not receive breastmilk, who otherwise will be at risk of increasing malnutrition and death.

The global headquarters of both WHO and Nestlé are situated in Switzerland, only fifty-six miles apart on the banks of Lake Geneva. Yet despite their geographical proximity they are not able to come together and agree a collective approach to the delivery of the best nutrition for infants and young children worldwide. The fact that they are both located in one of the most beautiful and affluent areas in the world – and the impact of their perceived dysfunctional behaviour is most deeply felt in the poorest areas in the world, generates further disquiet over their unprofessional behaviour.

WHO working with health professionals

Health professionals recognize that to provide the best nutritional care for their child patients there will be circumstances when good clinical practice involves consulting with industry, which may lead to discussions on collaborative research. It is also recognized that as nutritional care is a key element of all aspects of paediatric practice, multidisciplinary training and education on infant and child nutrition is an essential part of professional development. However, WHO have expressed concern about paediatricians collaborating with the infant-formula industry on research and education activities and have asserted that this is a conflict of interest for paediatricians.[6]

Partnership-working is a key element of many aspects of paediatric care, however it has proved problematic in infant and child nutrition. WHO not only adopts a policy of non-cooperation with the infant and young child food industry, but also takes measures to restrict contact with industry by other partners. This approach simply magnifies the issues and ignores the widely held view that the key to conflict resolution is communication.

The position of WHO seems to be that they do not see the infant-formula industry as a partner and they do not trust them sufficiently to participate in discussions on policy, research, training and education.[1] Furthermore, WHO do not trust health professionals to be able to resist any commercial pressure that industry may or may not impose upon them (as inferred from published correspondence and articles).

In 2016 WHO took the unusual step of criticizing the Royal College of Paediatrics and Child Health (RCPCH) through the columns of *The Lancet*, because the College was continuing to accept funding from infant-formula companies to support their annual meeting, which provides educational opportunities for their members who provide paediatric care in most countries worldwide.[6] The WHO accused the RCPCH of creating competing interests. The College responded that with respect to engagement with industry, including infant-formula companies, the revisions to their long-standing policy were agreed by the RCPCH Council in October 2016, after a detailed membership consultation process that provided a strong majority mandate. In brief, the RCPCH's policy for accepting donations encourages donors, including infant-formula manufacturers – subject to due diligence – to contribute to funds that support activities that benefit infants, children and young people. Donations from industry are transparent and acknowledged, and they do not permit the involvement of industry, or the linking of a name or logo, to any specific output.[7]

It is most unfortunate that WHO officials took the path of trying to undermine the reputation of paediatricians in a public statement, which was strong on surmise and weak on material evidence. The RCPCH has more than 20,000 members and for WHO criticisms to have any credence they need to provide information on the number of paediatricians who have been found guilty of criminality or professional misconduct in relation to their association with industry. And if they did have evidence of misconduct, there are regulatory systems in place that enable formal investigations of such allegations.

The core issue underpinning this altercation and other similar claims relates to differing perceptions of what is, or what is not, consistent with the recommendations contained within the Code. Although WHO claim that the RCPCH (and therefore paediatricians worldwide) are failing to abide by the Code, it is noted that a paediatrician's duty of care primarily relates to the clinical needs of their child patients. There will be situations in which decisions need to be made in the interest of a patient rather than the Code.

With the priority for the paediatrician being the health and wellbeing of their patients a commitment to maintaining skills and knowledge is essential. It is unfortunate that WHO and breastfeeding activist groups have interpreted any contact with industry on educational or research matters, as a conflict of interest and have used the Code as a tool to undermine the reputation and commitment of paediatricians and other health professionals. A key objective of the Code is to encourage cooperation between all stakeholders in order to improve the health and wellbeing of children worldwide. The action of the WHO officials clearly conflicts with the ethos of effective partnership-working. Moreover, expecting compliance with a document developed for the 1980s, to still be compliant in the 2020s, and to not have been updated in the meantime, lacks credibility and basic governance, especially when no country is fully compliant after forty years and only 12.7% of countries have been classified as substantially compliant.[8] With the current statistics showing that the annual increase in global substantial compliance is 0.32% per year, if the ambition is to achieve 100 % compliance, progress at this rate it will take more than a hundred years. It is therefore evident that acceptable levels of compliance will only be achieved if the Code is reviewed by all stakeholders and consensus is achieved on the key disputed areas of the Code. Planning a strategy without involving the key individuals or groups who will have responsibility for delivery of the strategy, will inevitably result in low compliance.

The authors of the WHO letter to *The Lancet* are senior officials within WHO, and the letter makes several references to the WHO Code and WHA resolutions, yet there is a declaration at the end of the letter that states:

"The authors alone are responsible for the views expressed in this letter and they do not necessarily represent the views, decisions, or policies of WHO".

They also declared that they have 'no competing interests'.[6] They clearly support the WHO resolutions with which they are closely involved, and they are presumably remunerated by WHO for their employment. It is therefore difficult to understand how they have 'no competing interests'. If the letter was from four employees of a large pharmaceutical company, complaining that paediatricians were not prescribing their new fully licensed antibiotic, and the authors signed off the letter with a declaration of no competing interests, would this not be considered a serious material conflict of interest?

On 13 February 2019, following a Council decision, the RCPCH declared that it would no longer accept any further funding from formula-milk companies, but it will continue to receive funding from other sources. The College did state that specialist formula milks are crucial for protecting the health, and in many cases their lives, of infants who cannot breastfeed. These milks are prescribed by paediatricians and can be vital for pre-term babies, young children with allergies or gastrointestinal conditions, and those whose mothers cannot breastfeed.[9]

The RCPCH also stated that it will maintain its due diligence process in respect of all corporate relationships, through which it will seek to influence formula-milk companies' marketing behaviours around the world; and it will continue regularly to engage with them in order to further improve communication and understanding. The RCPCH resolutely believes that through this engagement it will generate the best opportunity to improve the health and wellbeing of infants and young children.

They also clarified that funding research into specialist formula milks by a formula-milk company, that is carried out in an academic or clinical institution under its own due diligence, and from which salaries are drawn, is not in any way affected by this statement. They also stated that any health professional can accept funding from formula-milk companies to attend an event at which 'scientific and factual information' is shared. This is enshrined in WHO Code Article 7.5.

The intervention and the language used by WHO officials in their letter to *The Lancet* indicate that they have a different attitude to partnership-working with industry compared to their WHO colleagues who have responsibility for epidemic/pandemic preparedness. Following the Ebola epidemic, the lessons learnt included the need for closer partnership-working with industry to develop diagnostic tests, vaccines and medicines to prevent the virus and treat subsequent infections. The learning from these lessons was apparent in the Covid-19 pandemic, whereby industry was strongly encouraged to provide diagnostic tests, vaccines and treatments as soon as possible. And, of course, health professionals were on the frontline of the pandemic, placing their own lives at risk, many of whom lost their lives providing care to their patients. The public denouncement of commitment and integrity of health professionals in the columns of *The Lancet* was a damaging misjudgement from the WHO officials.

All research, training and educational activities require funding, and the issue of sponsorship can be challenging. The potential benefits of improving knowledge and skills must be carefully balanced against the risks of potential conflicts of interest. With partnership-working enabling a greater sense of trust as well as closer alignment in strategic direction, the assessment of benefit versus risk can be undertaken with due diligence. If the conditions of the sponsorship are met, and there is transparency in the decision-making process, with audit of the outcome, then the sponsorship can be justifiably accepted on the grounds that it will serve the best interests of children and their health professionals.

Partnerships strengthen governance, and the failure to accommodate industry in a partnership provides a continuing source of conflict and mistrust. Whether it is industry or another member of the partnership that steps out of line, it is the responsibility of the other partners to take appropriate action. The effectiveness of a partnership can be strengthened by the adoption of shared principles such as integrity, solidarity, justice, equality, and cooperation all of which can be achieved with effective leadership.[10]

A Strategic Advisory Group (SAG) on infant and young-child feeding

I believe that as part of the development of its partnership structure and process, WHO needs to strengthen relations with a wider range of contributors to infant-feeding research, policy and practice and ensure that their outputs are more representative of the wider infant-feeding community. Their policies need to address infant-feeding issues, especially those relating to the most vulnerable populations, with manageable incremental improvements. This may require policy statements that do not initially meet idealistic aspirations but will, through effective engagement, set a path of improvement for those infants and young children with the greatest need.

The SAG should be independent of WHO/WHA structures and appropriately represented to provide the right perspective on strategic priorities and aspirations.

It should also be viewed as providing an element of independent governance around policy strategy, and should ensure that policy decisions are not overly influenced by internal preferences, prejudices or external politics. The group would be independent, providing an advisory role to the WHO Secretariat and Executive Board and WHA.

References

1. Branca F, Demaio A, Udomkesmalee E, *et al.* (2020) A new nutrition manifesto for a new nutrition reality. *The Lancet* 395, 8–10.

2. ILSI Europe. Website homepage. Available at: https://ilsi.eu/ (last accessed August 2022).

3. Forsyth S (2012) FTSE, WHO Code and the infant-formula industry. *Annals of Nutrition and Metabolism* 60, 154–56. DOI: 10.1159/000337304.

4. *Access to Nutrition Index* (2018) Available at: https://accesstonutrition.org/app/uploads/2020/02/GI_Global-Index_Full_Report_2018.pdf.

5. WHO/UN Children's Fund (2017) *NetCode toolkit. Monitoring the marketing of breastmilk substitutes: protocol for ongoing monitoring systems.* Licence CC BY-NC-SA 3.0 IGO. Available at: https://apps.who.int/iris/bitstream/handle/10665/259441/9789241513180-eng.pdf (last accessed August 2022).

6. Costello A, Branca F, Rollins N, *et al.* (2017) Health professional associations and industry funding. *The Lancet* 389, 597.

7. Modi N, Greenough A, Viner R, *et al.* for the Royal College of Paediatrics and Child Health (2017) RCPCH statement on future funding agreements with formula milk companies. *The Lancet* 389, 1693. Available at: https://www.rcpch.ac.uk/news–events/news/rcpch–statement–future–funding–agreements–formula–milk–companies/ (last accessed August 2022).

8. Forsyth S (2021) 40th anniversary of the *International Code of Marketing of Breastmilk Substitutes. The Lancet* 398, 1042.

9. RCPH (2019) *RCPCH supplementary statement and FAQs on formula milk.* Available at: https://www.rcpch.ac.uk/news-events/news/rcpch-supplementary-statement-faqs-formula-milk (last accessed August (2022).

10. Singh JA, Daar AS, Singer PA (2010) Principles of ethics for infant and young-child nutrition in the developing world. *BMC Public Health* 10, 321.

CHAPTER 14

Product regulation
and monitoring

The aim of the International Code was to contribute to the provision of safe and adequate nutrition for infants, by the protection and promotion of breastfeeding, and by ensuring the proper use of breastmilk substitutes, when these are necessary, on the basis of adequate information and through appropriate marketing and distribution.[1]

However, despite the introduction of the Code and many subsequent measures by WHO and other organizations, violations of the Code continue to be reported and concerns have been raised about potential health consequences worldwide.[2] The infant-formula industry is considered to be the *bête noir* of the infant-feeding community, which reflects a long history of marketing and promotional activities that have not been compliant with the Code. The continuing controversy surrounding non-compliance has had a negative impact on partnership-working, with increasing acrimony and division across the key stakeholders.[3]

Unfortunately, this conflict within the policy-making process has been allowed to continue for four decades, reflecting not only a lack of trust and respect within the infant-feeding community but also an absence of an independent regulatory authority. It is important that the passage of infant-formula products, from development within industry to purchase by parents in the community, is closely monitored and regulated to make sure parents are appropriately informed and their infants are adequately protected.

Violations committed by industry most commonly relate to the product not meeting Code recommendations on marketing, promotion, labelling and packaging. Additionally, there have been issues regarding the optimum nutritional composition of infant formulas, and achieving consensus may be difficult, even across national, regional and global authorities, including EFSA, the US FDA and the Codex Alimentarius Commission, which has global responsibility for assessing the validity and safety of infant-formula composition.

Evaluation of changes in formula composition

Research that leads to the proposal of an additional nutrient for infant formulas needs to be closely examined to ensure the evidence is robust and the product is safe. It is not surprising that health authorities such as WHO and breastfeeding interest groups want to ensure that if an infant formula is required, that any change to composition will provide additional health benefit, and is not simply a marketing ploy by industry to increase sales.

It is also important for infants who are not breastfed that self-interest does not result in formula-fed infants being further disadvantaged. Every effort should be made to provide them with a formula that most closely meets their nutritional requirements, however, there have been circumstances when there has been resistance to the introduction of new nutrients to formulas. Although it is important to be satisfied with the scientific evidence, it should also be obligatory for decisions not to be influenced by anti-industry sentiments. The most high-profile case in which the interests of scientists, industry and civil society clashed over an issue of formula composition relates to the addition of the long-chain PUFA called DHA, to standard infant formulas. The decision process led all the way to the European Parliament.

DHA and infant formulas

DHA is an omega-3 long-chain PUFA that is rapidly taken up by the infant brain and retina between twenty weeks' gestation and two years of age. Over the last three decades there has been considerable research interest in the potential role DHA may have in infant cognitive and visual development. A number of factors indicate DHA is important for the developing infant:

- There is an active transport mechanism for DHA crossing the placenta from mother to infant, resulting in higher blood levels in the infant compared to the mother.
- Maternal dietary intake of oily fish increases levels of DHA in breastmilk.
- Breastmilk samples have been tested worldwide showing that DHA is always present in breastmilk.
- DHA concentrations in the infant brain are higher in breastfed infants compared to those fed formulas without added DHA.
- There are published studies indicating that formulas with added DHA improve visual and cognitive function.

In 2008, based on the published evidence linking DHA to visual development, Mead Johnson Nutritionals, a US manufacturer of infant formulas (including those containing DHA) applied for a health claim to the EFSA pursuant to Article 14 (EC Regulation No 1924/2006). The EFSA has responsibility for improving food safety within the EU. As a risk assessor, it produces scientific opinion and advice to the European Commission, European Parliament and EU member states. Within EFSA, the Panel on Dietetic Products, Nutrition and Allergies addresses questions relating to dietetic products, nutrition and food allergies, as well as associated issues such as novel foods.

At that time, the panel had a membership of twenty-one risk-assessment experts from a number of European nations with expertise in a range of relevant fields. Appointments were made on the basis of proven scientific excellence following an open call for applications and a rigorous selection procedure. All experts working for EFSA signed a declaration of interests to safeguard EFSA's commitment to independence.

In the Mead Johnson application, the health claim related to the contribution of DHA to optimal visual development of infants and young children (from birth to three years of age). The applicant identified a total of forty-three publications, including thirteen randomized controlled trials (RCTs). On the basis of the data presented, the EFSA panel concluded that a 'cause and effect' relationship had been established between the intake of infant formula and follow-on formula supplemented with DHA and visual development in early life.[4]

Before final authorization by the European Commission was granted, the opinion of EFSA was challenged by the UK-based activist group Baby Milk Action, who initiated a campaign to have the decision reversed. Although Baby Milk Action has a track record of campaigning against infant-formula companies, on this occasion they were questioning the scientific integrity and competence of EFSA. Effective lobbying resulted in a group of Members of the European Parliament (MEPs), led by UK MEP Glenys Willmott, submitting a resolution that opposed the adoption of the health claim.[5] The arguments set out in the resolution included the assertion that:

- the biological environment for DHA in formulas is different from that of breastmilk
- a systematic review had not reported benefit from added DHA[6]
- there is a need for more research into the possible beneficial and harmful effects
- there is not a clear scientific consensus.

The resolution was considered by the European Parliament's Committee on Environment, Public Health and Food Safety on 16 March 2011. The resolution aimed to refuse authorization of the health claim, and was adopted (thirty votes in favour, twenty-eight against and one abstention). Following this, procedure dictated that the resolution was to go before the full European Parliament, which took place on the 6 April 2011.

The outcome of that vote was that the resolution opposing authorization did not achieve the necessary qualified majority of votes (three hundred and eighty-eight), so it was not passed. The vote was three hundred and twenty-eight votes in favour and three hundred and twenty-three against, with twenty-six abstentions.

The voting reflected political party lines, whereby social democratic and green parties voted for the resolution, and conservatives against. The vote meant that Mead Johnson's claim, that DHA intake contributed to the normal visual development of infants up to twelve months of age, was able to enter the EU legislature.

The reaction to the outcome of the vote tended to reflect the political perspectives. The response from Baby Milk Action was that authorization of the claim handed industry the marketing tool they desired – and brought the important process relating to health claims into disrepute. A representative from industry stated that science, innovation and choice prevailed, and that the vote reinforced the scientific independence and credibility of the EU food safety and health-claims system.

Julie Girling, a UK Conservative MEP, defended the right of manufacturers to make such claims and added that denying this information on the grounds that mothers are not fit to make decisions for themselves is an example of the overbearing EU 'nanny state' at its worst. Glenis Willmott commented that what is in the best interests of a multinational's marketing department might not be in the best interests of parents. In a letter to Glenis Willmott, the WHO said:

"WHO does not have a recommendation about the addition of [DHA] to formula milk … to date no solid evidence exists to be able to say that adding DHA to infant formula will have important clinical benefits. Were WHO to give such a recommendation, it would have to follow a strict guideline development process based on grading of all available evidence collected through systematic reviews by expert panels free from conflict of interest".

This WHO comment is interesting from two perspectives:

- First, they have continued to be resistant to the addition of DHA and ARA to infant formulas, despite accumulating research evidence and the presence of these fatty acids in breastmilk.

- Second, they are publicly questioning the integrity and competence of the EFSA scientific assessment.
- Third, they clearly do not apply such rigorous standards to their own recommendations on infant-feeding policy, such as the re-defining of breastmilk substitute.

Expert panels on infant-formula composition that are free from conflict of interest are difficult to establish if collaboration with industry is viewed as a conflict of interest. Undertaking interventional nutrition clinical studies to investigate a specific nutrient is not possible without industry preparing the intervention products. Therefore, a panellist without previous collaboration with industry will not have experience of carrying out this type of study.

Finally, EFSA are highly respected for their strict governance standards and rigorous panel selection procedures. It may be that WHO's response is more reflective of their reluctance to co-function with industry.

The dubious situation of MEPs deciding whether a nutrient should be added to infant formulas and voting along political party lines is clearly incongruous. It reflects a lack of regulation and governance procedures overseeing infant-feeding policy-making. In 2021 the Codex Committee on Nutrition and Foods for Special Dietary Uses was in the final stages of reviewing a standard for infant formula and follow-up formula, including the requirement for DHA. It was recommended that DHA is provided as an *optional* ingredient for both infant and follow-up formulas, this Committee decision was not supported by WHO and breastfeeding interest groups.

Regulatory systems for marketing, promotion, labelling and packaging

NetCode

In 2014, WHO (in collaboration with UNICEF) established a Network for Global Monitoring and Support for Implementation of the Code and subsequent relevant WHA resolutions (NetCode).[7] Civil society member organizations include IBFAN, Helen Keller International, Save the Children Foundation, World Alliance for Breastfeeding Action and WHO Collaborating Centre at Metropol University. They state that their vision for NetCode is a world in which all sectors of society are protected from the inappropriate and unethical marketing of breastmilk substitutes and other products covered by the scope of the Code.

The goals are:

- to strengthen the capacity of member states and civil society to monitor the Code
- to facilitate the development, monitoring and enforcement of national Code laws by member states by bringing together a group of committed actors to support these processes.

When WHO in collaboration with IBFAN (and other breastfeeding interest groups) established this monitoring system, they clearly had not appreciated that the need was for an independent regulatory system. Their key objective is to monitor compliance with the Code and:

"… hold manufacturers, distributors, retail outlets, the healthcare system and healthcare workers to account for breaches of national laws and/or the Code"

And, when violations are alleged, they will encourage governments to impose sanctions as permitted by national legislation.

However, the organizations who initiated this process, and also participate as monitors, have a long history of preventing industry involvement in all aspects of infant-feeding policy and practice. Thus, they themselves have a material conflict of interest. NetCode is clearly divisive, with one half of the infant-feeding community monitoring the other half. There is not a reciprocal arrangement, and no reference is made to parents who are not activists but may have their own views on this matter.

FTSE4Good

In contrast to WHO, the infant-food industry has pursued systems in which there has been an attempt to provide an element of independent regulatory function. FTSE4Good was designed to act as a tool for investors who are interested in companies with acknowledged records of corporate social responsibility (including environmental sustainability, human rights and stakeholder involvement).[8] Following discussions with UNICEF, FTSE4Good established an index for companies that operate in the breastmilk substitute (BMS) sector, with the expectation that these companies will secure their inclusion in the FTSE4Good investment index by demonstrating that they meet specific marketing standards.[9,10] The FTSE4Good BMS Marketing Committee collaborated with an independent provider of research into company governance and ethical performance (the EIRIS Foundation) and developed BMS Marketing criteria that not only build on the Code and subsequent WHA resolutions, but also address the need for effective internal company-management systems. This process included consultation with companies, investors and NGOs, including both UNICEF UK and Save the Children.

If a BMS manufacturer meets the criteria to be included in the index, the company then undergoes an independent verification assessment to determine whether their practices on the ground follow their policies. PricewaterhouseCoopers (PwC) was appointed as the assessor for the first cycle of assessments, which were undertaken in two 'higher-risk' countries on the understanding that the risk of negative consequences from inappropriate marketing of BMS will be greatest in these countries. The criteria for defining a higher-risk country included rates of child malnutrition and child mortality. Using these criteria, a hundred and forty-nine countries were identified by FTSE. The plan was that FTSE would subsequently focus on activities in lower-risk countries. The infant-formula and food companies initially involved in the assessment phase included Abbott Laboratories, Danone, Heinz, Meiji Dairies, Pfizer and Nestlé.

In March 2011, Nestlé became the first company to meet the FTSE4Good selection criteria, which underwent a verification assessment of its practices in India and Zambia between April and August 2011. In a report from the Chief Executive of the FTSE Group to Nestlé on 14 November 2011, it was stated that 'on balance' Nestlé was meeting the criteria and had therefore maintained its position in the index.[11] However, there were aspects of policy and practice that Nestlé needed to address and these were to be reviewed during further verification assessments in 2012. Nestlé subsequently maintained its position on the index and, in 2016, was joined by Danone. The reactions of stakeholders and observers to this new initiative reflected a mix of encouragement, caution and suspicion.[12] However, FTSE, EIRIS and PwC have global reputations for the assessment of performance, ethics and audit within business, and their expertise will undoubtedly enhance the scrutiny of policies and practices in the infant-formula industry. FTSE emphasizes that the initiative is an evolutionary process, with the key components of engagement, gaining trust and continuous improvement.

The credibility of the initiative will largely depend on the robustness of the verification assessment. Correspondence from the FTSE Chief Executive to IBFAN clearly indicates that the verification is against the FTSE4Good criteria, not against the Code *per se* (see a summary of this correspondence in the *Addendum* to this chapter).[12] The Chief Executive indicates that the assessors will not act as a judge on specific allegations but will restrict their audit to assessing whether practices on the ground are in line with company policy. For assurance on the rigour of the assessment, the verification tool and the final report of all verification assessments are made available in the public domain.

With one hundred and forty-nine countries now identified to be at high risk, the selection of only two countries to determine whether a company is meeting the set criteria may raise doubts about the comprehensiveness and validity of the assessment.

It has also been suggested that a larger representation at the initial verification assessment, with fewer countries involved as spot checks at subsequent assessments, may provide greater assurance on the overall performance of the company. The countries are currently selected by a risk-assessment matrix devised by the auditors, PwC and the BMS Expert Committee.

With the effectiveness of the Code having hitherto been undermined by longstanding self-regulatory failure, this FTSE initiative should be viewed as an opportunity to strengthen the Code with governance structures that are robust and independent. The initiative is, however, still at an early stage of development and for it to be sustainable it will not only require a substantive and transparent commissioning process but also commitment from key stakeholders across the infant-feeding community. It is uncertain whether FTSE4Good sees this initiative as a long-term commitment.

Access to Nutrition Index (ANI)

The *Access to Nutrition Index* (ANI) was initially launched in 2013 and has a sub-ranking for breastmilk-substitute companies who joined the Index in 2016.[13] Six manufacturers of breastmilk substitutes were assessed using a separate additional BMS methodology. The criteria applied to select these manufacturers was that they needed to be manufacturers of breastmilk substitutes, and baby-food sales had to account for more than 5% of their total sales in 2013. Four food and beverage (F&B) sector companies were included on this basis, along with the two largest manufacturers of infant formula and baby foods. Alignment of company policies with the 1981 Code was assessed, as was the quality of management systems used to implement those policies and their disclosure of policies and practices. In addition, the companies' marketing practices in the capital cities of Indonesia and Vietnam were assessed by Westat, an independent research organization, using the Interagency Group on Breastfeeding Monitoring (IGBM) protocol. In 2021, Danone led the BMS marketing sub-ranking with an overall score of 68%, having scored 46% in 2018 and 31% in 2016. Next comes Nestlé with 57%, an improvement from 45% in 2018 and 31% in 2016.

So, at present there are three systems in place that are assessing compliance with the Code by breastmilk-substitute companies, none of which has the undivided support of the most vocal stakeholders (see the correspondence in Boxes 14.1–14.4 in the *Addendum* to this chapter). With the history of deep-seated, longstanding divisions it is unlikely that any form of assessment will meet the wishes of WHO, industry and breastfeeding interest groups. In the meantime, global compliance with the Code remains poor.[14]

Transformational change

A key finding from each of these systems is that obtaining reliable and complete information during the in-market period is geographically challenging when there are one hundred and ninety-seven countries worldwide. A system that depends on country visits to identify evidence of failure to comply with Code recommendations is unlikely to be viable in the long-term. Saying that, the above data show that infant-formula companies do appear to be responding in a positive way to initiatives that are aimed at improving their compliance with the Code. This progress should be acknowledged and, as the Chief Executive of FTSE commented:

> "… it is an important act of trust to allow a third party to undertake an independent assessment of your operations".

It is likely that some of the other stakeholders would be reluctant to subject their operations to such an investigation by an external body. Although some of them will remain sceptic, the incremental improvement by the companies, as measured by the independent assessors, should be perceived as evidence that attitudes and behaviours of infant-formula companies can be changed, and that it should be possible to build on the experience of FTSE4Good and ANI to create a system that has good outreach and is adequately regulated.

The issues of visits for assessment include:

- technical difficulties in arranging unannounced visits
- the choice of venues that may not reflect other parts of the country
- retrospective information not being as robust and trustworthy as data collected prospectively
- the validity of judgements on infant-feeding practice across an entire country or region based on a short visit by observers.

As a consequence of these uncertainties, the outcomes of visits and the quality of evidence tend to be challenged, which creates yet more acrimony and division.

The model adopted by each of these systems appears to be 'back-to-front'. Products are allowed to enter the global market without a robust official assessment of their compliance with the Code in relation to marketing, promotion, labelling and packaging during the pre-market period, and evidence of non-compliance is subsequently investigated across the multinational global market. This is clearly a time-consuming, labour-intensive, ineffective and costly process.

In contrast, a system that applies a robust pre-market assessment of all infant-formula products before they enter the open market could be more efficient, more sustainable and more cost-effective. More than this, the existence of a prospective database of all products that have been authorized worldwide prior to entering the market will provide a valuable source of background evidence for investigating future claims of violations of the Code made during the in-market period. Rather than undertaking at most two site visits per year, technological solutions for collecting global data should be considered (such as the use of smart phones and other digital technology), which should allow global data to be collected online and provide real-time communication between parents, health professionals and other relevant groups.

Pre-market assessment of infant formula products

The underlying principles of a new system should be that a formula will not be released to the global market until a thorough pre-market assessment is completed and a seal of approval is given. The key objectives of the new system should be:

- it will reduce non-compliance
- it has capability to provide a global workable solution
- it can provide violation data relating to specific products, companies and countries
- it is underpinned by key governance and regulatory procedures
- there is a commitment and endorsement from all key stakeholders.

The assessment will need to be comprehensive and consistent for all products, with evaluations of all relevant marketing and promotion materials (Fig. 14.1). Only after this intensive assessment of the submitted materials can it be concluded that the evidence meets nationally and globally agreed standards, and the formula and related materials can be authorized and registered. Materials not included in this assessment cannot be subsequently used in marketing and promotion without making a further submission to the relevant trading standards authority. The seal of approval will be available on both the product and the related authorized literature and other materials, which should include online contact details for consumers and other interested parties that confirms that authorization and registration of the product has been obtained. The products on the shelves of retailers without a seal of approval, or with unauthorized information, would be non-compliant and the retailers and/or manufacturers held culpable. This process should be considered a global standard and validation system that applies to all current infant-formula companies worldwide, and any new companies that join the market. Different regions may adopt different processes, but there should be agreement on key assessment measures that will provide a minimum global standard, with such data held on the global register.

This system will be measurable because all trading standards institutions will have agreed the core minimum standards that apply to all companies and their infant-formula products worldwide. The information will be available on an accessible global register. By creating a system through which parents, health professionals or any other organizations or individuals can select a product off the shelf, at any location worldwide, and use their smart phone to digitally contact the authorization centre to check the authorization status of the product, to read the relevant material, and to view images of the products. This will provide immediate reassurance that the product is compliant with the Code. Furthermore, if parents or other individuals have concerns about the validity of a product, there will be guidance about the seal of approval and on how to report a possible violation. A real-time information system like this, as well as providing assurance to parents, will also convey a warning message to any manufacturer or retailer that the inappropriate marketing of a product is far more likely to be detected, and that the consequences will be significant, including suspension of the product.

With most infant-formula companies serving global markets, there can be allegations of Code violation occurring in one country, while the company headquarters are located in another country, and the trading standards centre in yet another country. For this reason, any global system must ensure that the assessment processes and investigations of allegations of non-compliance can be conducted across country, regional and continental boundaries.

Partnership-working

The cooperation of industry is essential and, collectively, companies need to adopt a responsible and ethical approach to the marketing and promotion of infant-formula products. The new system would provide hard data on the abuse of marketing and promotion at a global level, which will initiate appropriate regulatory action. If regulation of the system is unsuccessful, then formal legislation will be required. This will hopefully be viewed by industry as an opportunity, not only to settle forty years of conflict with WHO on Code matters, but also to see that this proposal clarifies the rules regarding authorization and provides a level playing field for all participants. With violations relating to inappropriate marketing and promotion by industry leading to collateral criticism and restrictions on healthcare professionals and parents by WHO, the potential benefits of a more focused and effective system of control should lead to more constructive partnership-working in the future.

Codex Alimentarius

The Codex Alimentarius Commission has a global responsibility for protecting the health of consumers and ensuring fair practices in the international food trade.[15] Through their Committee on Nutrition and Food for Special Dietary Uses, the organization has developed global standards for infant formulas, follow-up formulas and complementary foods. It is therefore proposed that Codex is the lead organization for ensuring that breastmilk substitutes are appropriately assessed and authorized and maintains the global register for access by any relevant party to ensure a specific product meets all agreed composition and presentation standards. A Codex office should be the point of contact for national and regional trading standards offices that have responsibility for authorizing infant-formula products and related materials.

The process should be underpinned by a digital communication system that is interactive and can be elaborated on to become publicly accessible. There will need to be strong and decisive leadership to bring key stakeholders together, to enable the process to develop and potential benefits to emerge. To strengthen the governance of this system an independent advisory body should be appointed that will undertake an annual review of the process, consider the data on compliance and violations, and make recommendations for further development.

In conclusion, a transformational change in the monitoring, marketing and promotion of infant formulas is proposed. It consists of a robust pre-market regulation system that is underpinned by agreed global standards, with a global register of authorizations, and through digital technology provides real-time access and feedback to consumers and other interested parties worldwide. The overall responsibility for this system might rest with the Codex Alimentarius Commission, as this organization has global responsibility for protecting

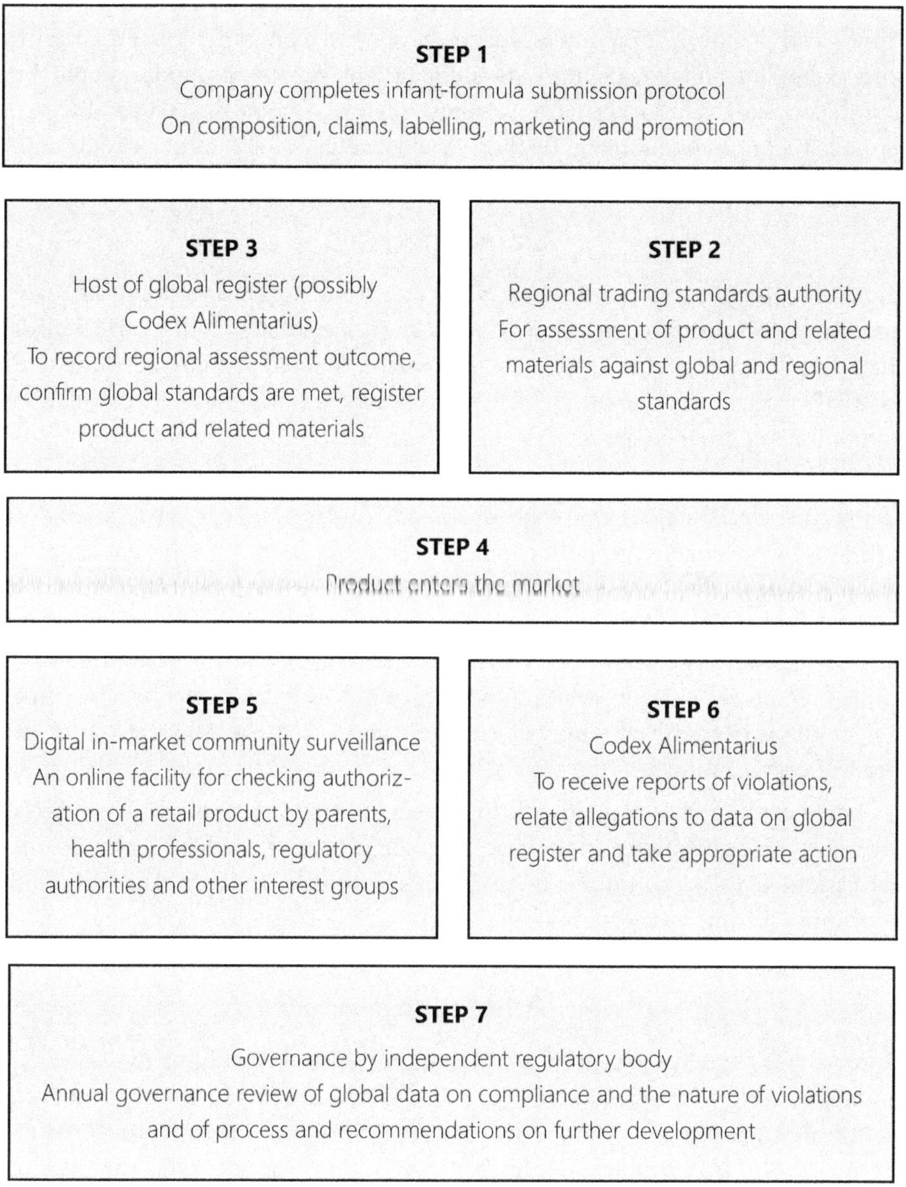

STEP 1
Company completes infant-formula submission protocol
On composition, claims, labelling, marketing and promotion

STEP 3
Host of global register (possibly
Codex Alimentarius)
To record regional assessment outcome,
confirm global standards are met, register
product and related materials

STEP 2
Regional trading standards authority
For assessment of product and related
materials against global and regional
standards

STEP 4
Product enters the market

STEP 5
Digital in-market community surveillance
An online facility for checking authorization of a retail product by parents,
health professionals, regulatory
authorities and other interest groups

STEP 6
Codex Alimentarius
To receive reports of violations,
relate allegations to data on global
register and take appropriate action

STEP 7
Governance by independent regulatory body
Annual governance review of global data on compliance and the nature of violations
and of process and recommendations on further development

Fig. 14.1: Proposed global regulatory structure for submission, assessment, authorization and monitoring of infant formulas and related materials.

consumers and ensuring fair trade. It is already responsible for assessing infant-formula composition, and makes recommendations on nutrition and health claims, labelling and packaging. An independent regulatory body should be appointed to undertake an annual governance review of global data on compliance and make recommendations on further developments.

Conclusion

Product regulation and monitoring is always going to be a contentious area if there is a lack of agreement on what is the acceptable standard. If there is underlying disagreement on policy statements contained within the Code and also WHO's infant and young-child feeding policy, the standards for regulating and monitoring progress are always going to be questioned.

It is evident that governance systems cannot be considered in isolation to policy and practice decisions so there needs to be a collective approach involving continuity between science, policy, practice and regulation. At present there is friction between all of these key stages of product development and delivery, which undoubtedly adds to the difficulty and frustration experienced by the influential global organizations FTSE4Good and PwC who have attempted to establish regulatory systems relating to the Code. This must surely be a learning point, perhaps even a 'wake-up call' for the hierarchy of WHO/WHA and the other UN organizations.

The primary function of regulation is to protect those individuals who are subject to decisions made by others. In the case of infant feeding, the 'others' have become so accustomed to making their own rules; the idea of collective thinking and compromise is difficult for them to process.

Addendum

The correspondence between FTSE, Nestlé and IBFAN highlight the differing opinions relating to the role of FTSE as they attempt to provide a regulatory function in a challenging – and at times hostile – environment. Here I provide a summary of the key issues identified by the individual parties at the time of the initial assessments in 2011–2012 (Boxes 14.1–14.4). FTSE supported the idea that the correspondence was available within the public domain, in its entirety. The relevant online links are provided, together with key extracts of the correspondence.

Box 14.1: Extracts of a letter from the Chief Executive of FTSE to the Chief Executive of Nestlé SA (14 November 2011)

Source: https://research.ftserussell.com/products/downloads/ftse_letter_to_ nestle.pdf/.

- **Extract 1.** "It is an important act of trust to allow a third party to undertake an independent assessment of your operations. I therefore wanted to thank you for agreeing to this verification. Your colleagues have worked diligently and transparently with both ourselves and PwC and I wanted to record our appreciation of this. In addition I wanted to provide you with a summary of the key findings and next steps."

- **Extract 2.** "A significant issue is the 'boundaries of responsibility'. The FTSE4Good Criteria requires no promotion of BMS products in high-risk countries. In order to achieve this it requires manufacturers to work closely with their distributors and retailers to ensure that these organizations are aware of the company's policies. This can be a challenging task. A parallel can be drawn with supply-chain labour standards in ensuring that suppliers, sometimes multiple steps removed from the company, are meeting labour standards. On this topic many companies, including Nestlé, have taken responsibility for the actions of their suppliers and found approaches to influence and to a large extent ensure minimum standards are met. We recognize that influencing a distribution chain can be more challenging than a supply chain, not least because there are anti-trust and other commercial laws that affect this. However the assessment did identify that in one of the countries visited there were cases of inappropriate promotional activities by retailers selling Nestlé BMS products. The Committee would like to see a clearer policy and stronger implementation in order to ensure retailers and distributors are aware of Nestlé's policy regarding the marketing and promotion of BMS products in high-risk countries."

- **Extract 3.** "Certain marketing practices, including the use of specialist display cabinets for BMS products in Zambia, could be regarded as promotional. In addition, there were some questions raised by the BMS Committee regarding conference attendance for healthcare professionals in India. Arguments can be made regarding the scientific and educational benefits of supporting conference attendance, but it raises questions on the extent to which this could be regarded as a promotional activity. Whilst these may be regarded as grey areas, the Committee would like Nestlé to analyze these practices, and to consider more broadly what is regarded as promotional."

- **Extract 4.** "The assessment indicated that only a Nutrition Code-Compliance Manager and a Public Affairs Manager received the annual summary reports on internal monitoring, external reporting and corrective actions regarding BMS marketing activities. As stated in the FTSE4Good BMS Marketing Criteria, the Committee noted that Nestlé's Group Board of Directors must receive these reports and would like to know Nestlé's intent on this matter."

- **Extract 5.** "Many of the Nestlé policies and reports on BMS marketing were difficult to find online and transparency should be improved by making these documents easier to locate. In addition, the Committee would like clarification on whether the Nestlé 'ombudsman process' will be able to involve independent investigation of issues raised, and the Committee would like to see some examples to demonstrate that the whistleblowing procedures are effective."

- **Extract 6.** "Next steps are that Nestlé should respond to these points and the BMS Marketing Committee (a sub-committee of the Policy Committee) would like to hear of any plans or future policies that would address them. It was noted that the next reviews of the Index will be in March and September 2012, when the Committee will meet again and review Nestlé's on-going inclusion."

Box 14.2: Extracts from the response of the Chief Executive of Nestlé SA to the Chief Executive of FTSE (18 November 2011)

Source: https://research.ftserussell.com/products/downloads/Nestlé_Letter_ of_Response.pdf/.

- **Extract 1.** "We have appreciated the opportunity to work with FTSE in the process of your evaluation of our breastmilk-substitute marketing policies, procedures and practices for inclusion in the FTSE4Good Index. This has enabled us to do further diligent review and reinforce our policy and systems for management of our compliance with WHO Code."

- **Extract 2.** "We are pleased to be the first and only breastmilk-substitute manufacturer which has been included in the FTSE4Good Index so far. We also appreciate the transparency with which FTSE has approached the evaluation and reporting. We would like to thank you for this and for allowing us to respond to your remarks identifying areas for improvement, which will be a helpful contribution to our continuing efforts to improve."

- **Extract 3.** "We recognize that third parties, or those even further removed from our direct distributors, sometimes carry out acts which are not consistent with our policies relative to WHO Code of Marketing of Breastmilk Substitutes, and this is an area of concern. We certainly want to find ways to bring to bear positive influence on those third parties at all levels but want to point out that this is a highly complex area. We make every effort to ensure that the distributors, importers, agents and retailers who are appointed by us and who buy our infant-nutrition products are informed about the requirements of WHO Code. Our policies and procedures provide that our written contracts with them in higher-risk countries include specific provisions about our WHO Code compliance policy. We provide them with information on what is and what is not allowed. When non-compliant point-of-sale activities are found, we contact the third party to remind them of the relevant requirements of WHO Code and the national Code (where there is one)."

- **Extract 4.** "The question of what is and what is not promotional is a discussion that has been ongoing since WHO Code was adopted in 1981, and we agree that there are grey areas. Nestlé has extensively described what we think is appropriate/not appropriate and shared this with the EIRIS, the FTSE Committees and posted it in the public domain. Whilst we feel that our approach takes a clear and strong position on promotional activities, we look forward to entering into discussions with you to see if there is any further action we can take to clarify our policies and procedures in this respect."

- **Extract 5.** "We regret that FTSE has experienced some difficulty in finding key documents related to our WHO Code compliance and we will take steps to ensure that the documents referred to are more easily accessible. We understand your comments on our ombudsman system. This system is intended to be a purely internal system for our own employees."

Box 14.3: IBFAN's concerns regarding the FTSE4Good Breastmilk Substitutes criteria, assessment process and BMS Committee (8 March 2012)

Source: http://info.babymilkaction.org/sites/info.babymilkaction.org/files/ IBFANtoFTSE%20080312.pdf/.

The response from IBFAN identified several concerns including the FTSE4Good assessment process, sponsorship and research, labelling, conflict of interest in the members of the BMS Committee and collaborators, and the FTSE4Good BMS Criteria.

- **Extract 1.** "FTSE provide a simple statement that can be used to counter misunderstandings and misrepresentation regarding FTSE4Good. Specifically, we ask FTSE to simply state that under the latest criteria and assessment process it is not necessary for a company to bring its marketing practices into line with the [Code] and subsequent relevant resolutions of the [WHA] or national laws implementing these measures to be included in the FTSE4Good Index."

- **Extract 2.** "The evidence available to us suggests that all breastmilk-substitute manufacturers currently violate the International Code routinely. We are therefore following the inclusion of Nestlé on the Index carefully and will be looking for evidence that their marketing begins to comply with the Code."

IBFAN specifically requested the following actions as a matter of urgency:

- *"The BMS Committee reconsiders its decision on Nestlé on the basis of the evidence provided and Nestlé's inadequate response.*
- *"The criteria for membership of the BMS Committee and its collaborators are reviewed to ensure that all members are free from conflicts of interest in relation to this issue.*
- *"The FTSE4Good criteria for assessment are reviewed to exclude companies that systematically violate the Code and subsequent WHA resolutions.*
- *"FTSE4Good writes to UNICEF HQ to request its opinion on the new FTSE criteria; to ask whether the Global Alliance for Improved Nutrition (GAIN) should be excluded from defining the procedures for including companies in the index; and to clarify the role of UNICEF UK and the appropriate use of the name UNICEF.*
- *"The Assessment Report of the monitoring is made public.*
- *"A clear statement is made that companies that systematically violate the Code and Resolutions can be included in the FTSE4Good Index under the current criteria and assessment criteria."*

Box 14.4: Extracts of a letter from the Chief Executive of FTSE to the Director of Policy at Baby Milk Action (13 March 2012)

Source: https://research.ftserussell.com/products/downloads/FTSE_Letter_to_Baby_Milk_Action_13.3.2012.pdf/.

- **Extract 1.** The criteria build on WHO Code by not only requiring policies to be aligned but through examining how effectively companies embed this into their governance, compliance systems and reporting. As you are aware, the FTSE4Good criteria are much more focused on company practices in higher-risk countries rather than low-risk countries, while WHO Code is universal in nature. In this respect the committee felt the weighting should be placed where there is the greatest risk to baby and infant lives and health, and that the tougher criteria could be expanded to cover the lower-risk countries over time. I accept that higher-risk regions exist in some lower-risk countries.
- **Extract 2.** The FTSE4Good BMS Marketing Committee concluded, using

the information from the independent verification assessment conducted by [PwC], that Nestlé was overall making good and reasonable efforts to implement its BMS marketing policies in the two 'high-risk' countries visited and hence was, on balance, meeting the criteria. Nestlé has therefore maintained its inclusion in the Index. However there were a number of areas that the FTSE4Good BMS Marketing Committee felt that Nestlé should improve, and we are in communication with Nestlé regarding these areas which are also set out publicly in my letter to Chief Executive of Nestlé. Again, this has been made available on our website.

- **Extract 3.** You raise concerns regarding the involvement of the Church of England, the Methodist Church and GAIN in our process and consultations. We find this surprising as these organizations all have a very strong focus on encouraging and catalyzing improved corporate practices and we have found their feedback extremely valuable. Most significant pension and investment schemes will have investments in global public equities, and it is not surprising that large investors such as the Church of England and the Methodist Church have Nestlé investments. Indeed, both organizations use their power as shareholders actively to influence investee companies (including Nestlé) to improve environmental, social and governance practices.

- **Extract 4.** FTSE strongly and actively supports the work of UNICEF through our longstanding corporate partnership with UNICEF UK. As I have mentioned previously neither UNICEF nor UNICEF UK are represented on the FTSE4Good BMS Committee. David Bull, the Executive Director of UNICEF UK, is an observer on the overall FTSE4Good Policy Committee which the FTSE4Good BMS Committee reports into. We have consulted widely over the BMS Marketing Criteria, including international organizations, NGOs and businesses.

- **Extract 5.** It is perhaps also worth noting that due to the high level of NGO interest we have placed much information on our website on this very specific topic that affects only eight companies from our assessment universe of over 2300 companies. Whilst we stand ready to provide more detailed information where this is beneficial, it is important that this is kept in context of the broader FTSE4Good inclusion criteria and assessment process for companies across all sectors.

- **Extract 6.** I know that you are disappointed with the decision over the two countries selected for the verification audit. We developed a country risk matrix with [PwC] and the BMS Committee and got advice from those we are collaborating with, which included NGOs and ethical investors. India and Zambia were selected as the outputs of the risk assessment matrix based on their high overall risk ratings, which were based on the wide variety of contributing risk factors in the risk-assessment matrix. The following factors were used to generate a risk score for each of the higher-risk countries in the FTSE4Good Inclusion Criteria: child mortality, malnutrition, access to improved water, access to midwives, corruption, human development, economic development, WHO member state, BMS regulation, IBFAN allegations, and scale of Nestlé activities.

- **Extract 7.** We appreciate that this is a sensitive topic and we have asked Nestlé to ensure that their references in communications regarding their inclusion in the FTSE4Good Series remain accurate and factual.

- **Extract 8.** We, and the Committee, feel that IBFAN has much to contribute to providing evidence into the verification process and before the verification assessment requested IBFAN support. I hope that you will be able to contribute to future assessments.

- **Extract 9.** As I have noted before, we feel that we have developed a robust process for what is a very sensitive and challenging issue. Other organizations providing ESG (environmental, social and governance) research and indices have usually avoided covering this topic due to the perceived controversy and challenges in developing realistic assessment methodologies. We hope to contribute to raising standards in this sector through raising awareness among investors and encouraging those companies who are prepared to make improvements to do so.

References

1. WHO (1981) *International Code of Marketing of Breastmilk Substitutes.* Geneva, WHO. Available at: extension://elhekieabhbkpmcefcoobjddigjcaadp/http://apps.who. int/iris/bitstream/handle/10665/40382/9241541601.pdf?sequence=1 (last accessed September 2022).

2. WHO (2016) *World Health Assembly resolution on the inappropriate promotion of foods for infants and young childre*n. Available at: https://apps.who.int/gb/ebwha/ pdf_files/WHA69/A69_R9-en.pdf?ua=1 (last accessed August 2022).

3. Forsyth JS (2010) *International Code of Marketing of Breastmilk Substitutes* – three decades later time for hostilities to be replaced by effective national and international governance. *Archives of Diseases in Childhood* 95, 769–70.

4. EFSA Scientific opinion (2009) DHA and ARA and visual development. Scientific substantiation of a health claim related to docosahexaenoic acid (DHA) and arachidonic acid (ARA) and visual development pursuant to Article 14 of EC Regulation No 1924/20061. Scientific Opinion of the Panel on Dietetic Products, Nutrition and Allergies (Question No EFSA-Q-2008–211). Adopted on 22 January 2009. *EFSA Journal* 941, 1–4.

5. Willmott G, Sarbu D, Childers N, Kadenbach K (2011) Motion for a resolution pursuant to Rule 88(2) of the Rules of Procedure by Glenis Willmott, Daciana Sarbu, Nessa Childers and Karin Kadenbach on the draft commission regulation on the authorisation and refusal of authorisation of certain health claims made on foods and referring to children's development and health. *European Parliament, Committee on the Environment, Public Health and Food Safety, Plenary Sitting B7 0000/2011.*

6. Simmer K, Patole SK, Rao SC (2008) Long-chain polyunsaturated fatty acid supplementation in infants born at term. *Cochrane Database of Systematic Reviews* CD000376.

7. WHO/UN Children's Fund (2017) *NetCode toolkit. Monitoring the marketing of breastmilk substitutes: protocol for ongoing monitoring systems. Licence CC BY-NC-SA 3.0 IGO.* Available at: https://apps.who.int/iris/bitstream/hand le/10665/259441/9789241513180-eng.pdf (last accessed August 2022).

8. FTSE Index Company (2011) *FTSE Group leads collaboration to improve breastmilk substitute marketing practices media information.* Available at: https://www.ftserussell. com/press/ftse-group-leads-collaboration-improve-breast-milk-substitute-marketing-practices (last accessed August 2022).

9. FTSE4Good (2011) *A note on the new FTSE4Good breastmilk substitute (BMS) marketing criteria and its impact on the FTSE4Good March 2011 Review.* Available at: https://research.ftserussell.com/products/downloads/FTSE4Good_Web_Update_ March_2011.pdf (last accessed August 2022).

10. FTSE4Good (2017) *Inclusion criteria for the marketing of breastmilk substitutes.* Available at: https://research.ftserussell.com/products/downloads/F4G_BMS_Criteria. pdf (last accessed August 2022).

11. *Letter from the Chief Executive, FTSE Group to Chief Executive Officer, Nestlé S.A.* (14 November 2011). Available at: https://research.ftserussell.com/products/ downloads/ftse_letter_to_nestle.pdf (last accessed August 2022).

12. *Letter to the Regional Coordinator, IBFAN, Asia* (17 June 2011). Available at: https:// research.ftserussell.com/products/downloads/letter_to_ibfan.pdf (last accessed August 2022).

13. *Access to Nutrition Index (2018)* Available at: https://accesstonutrition.org/app/ uploads/2020/02/GI_Global-Index_Full_Report_2018.pdf (last accessed August 2022).

14. WHO (2020) *Marketing of Breastmilk Substitutes: National Implementation of the International Code. Status Report 2020.* Available at: https://www.who.int/ publications/i/item/9789240006010 (last accessed August 2022).

15. Codex Alimentarius International Food Standards. Website homepage. Available at: https://www.fao.org/fao-who-codexalimentarius/publications/en/ (last accessed August 2022).

CHAPTER 15

Stakeholder conflict of interest and independent regulation

Many important developments in paediatric clinical care are the product of highly effective collaborations between researchers, clinicians and industry. As part of this, improvements in nutritional care have increased the survival of children struck by chronic illnesses with neonatal, metabolic, genetic, gastrointestinal and neurological conditions. However, in the area of infant and young-child nutrition within the general population, partnership-working, especially between WHO and the infant food industry, has a long history of acrimony and division. As a consequence, infant-feeding issues relating to policy and practice that were prominent more than four decades ago are still current today.[1]

The failure of WHO and industry to have a professional working relationship is a direct contravention of a key element of the Code that has been previously referenced, which states:

> *"… the need for governments, organizations of the United Nations system, non-governmental organizations, experts in various related disciplines, consumer groups and industry to cooperate in activities aimed at the improvement of maternal, infant and young-child health".[2]*

The divisions and mistrust continue and claims of conflict of interest are being used increasingly as a tool to undermine relations between stakeholders, especially if there is an interaction with industry. More recently, officials within WHO have turned their attention to the paediatric profession and made claims that specific aspects of their relationship with industry are a conflict of interest.[3]

It is interesting to note that although WHO and breastfeeding activists are proactive in holding to account other stakeholders who interact with industry, especially around the issue of inappropriate marketing of breastmilk substitutes, both WHO and industry tend to adopt similar behaviours in relation to their marketing and promotion of their respective products, breastmilk and infant formulas. For example:

- Both promote a nutritional product.
- Both tend to inappropriately market their product.

- Both tend to recruit stakeholders that are sympathetic to their beliefs and aspirations.
- Both tend to focus on their specific nutritional products, rather than take a holistic view of infant-feeding practice.
- Both lack independently agreed regulatory systems and independent governance standards.
- Both have been instrumental in creating decades of acrimony and division within the infant-feeding community.

It is therefore clear when considering conflict of interest and regulation, that the focus should be on all aspects of infant and young-child feeding, and no stakeholder should be exempt from critical appraisal.

Self-interest

The term 'self-interest' has occupied the minds of the world's greatest philosophers over many centuries, but whether self-interest is good or bad remains a topic of continuing debate. The term tends to be linked with financial gain, but in the example of someone deciding to pursue higher education in order to find a better job to obtain a higher income, it can reflect a positive attitude and provide motivation for personal and family betterment.

Similarly, scientific and healthcare staff who are committed to their profession may be motivated by self-interest to undertake specific areas of research in order to fulfil their desire to improve the quality of care for their patients, which may lead to financial and personal gain in terms of reputation, achievement and career opportunities. This scenario also applies to other groups including policymakers and parents.

Individuals with different self-interests may come together in a competitive or complementary way and provide overall benefit, as discussed by the eminent philosopher Adam Smith in the late eighteenth century, when he argued the case for 'division of labour' in his book *The Wealth of Nations*.[4] He stated that individuals, organizations, and nations are endowed with, or acquire, specialized capabilities that may include skills and training and various combinations of these assets; together they can produce outcomes that can provide a level of gain that is greater than the sum of the individual benefits.

These examples of self-interest and the associated potential benefits have to be considered when reflecting on the importance of partnership-working and how individual and collective self-interest can bring added value to policy decision-making. However the counterbalance is that, in some situations, self-interest can go beyond benefit and the abuse of self-interest leads to conflicts of interest, and potential harm and damage to the other partners and associates. In such circumstances a potential gain can revert to a destructive loss.

Conflict of interest

A conflict of interest within a healthcare environment has been defined as a set of circumstances by which a reasonable person would consider that an individual's ability to apply judgement or act, in the context of delivering healthcare services is, or could be, impaired or influenced by another interest they hold.[5] To be more precise, an *actual* conflict of interest can be defined as material conflict between one or more interests, and a *potential* conflict is the possibility of material conflict between one or more interests in the future. These interests are not restricted to financial benefits; they also include professional, personal and other indirect interests.

In relation to policymaking for infant feeding, many of the claims of conflict relate to a failure to abide by the recommendations set out in International Code, which was prepared by the WHO Secretariat and endorsed by the WHA in 1981. During the next forty years there has been no WHO/WHA-initiated review of the Code. As a consequence, there is now a new generation of parents, professionals and policymakers who have not had an opportunity to bring current thinking, knowledge or expertise to policy and practice relating to breastmilk substitutes.

In the meantime, WHO and WHA have taken the opportunity to change some aspects of the interpretation and meaning of the Code through intermittent 'resolutions'. It seems that WHO are protecting the Code by preventing the possibility of a review and are addressing any potential insurgency by inferring that it is driven by conflicts of interest. This situation would be described by the philosopher Adam Smith as a situation in which progress is being thwarted by those stakeholders who have assumed a position of dominance, and do not value the knowledge of others. Not surprisingly, the 'others' inevitably become demotivated, disengaged and distant.

Collaborative infant-feeding research

In a recent Editorial in the *British Medical Journal*, it was stated that paediatricians should disentangle themselves from 'Big Formula'.[5] But it is important to establish that nutrition intervention studies that are designed to determine optimum nutrient requirements for infants and young children cannot be undertaken without collaborating with nutrition companies. This is because the intervention product needs to meet established nutrition and safety standards, which requires knowledge, expertise and technology that is not available in even the most prestigious academic research institutions.[6] The days of scientists brewing up a concoction in their laboratory and administering it to research participants are long past.

It is also important in these collaborative intervention studies that industry is not considered a 'silent partner'. Their involvement should be as a full member of the research team, which ensures that their compliance with scientific, ethical, funding, and research monitoring standards are fully transparent. Moreover, all in-house research by industry should also be registered with an independent research trials registry, to make certain there is no suppression of any negative results. These standards should provide assurance that, on submission to a journal, the information regarding all of the contributors is complete, and the external reviewers and editorial team can then make an informed decision on whether to publish or not.

If this process is followed, and the article is accepted for publication, subsequent undermining of the research specifically on the grounds that it involved collaboration with industry should be challenged as professional discrimination. Although many paediatricians involved in infant-nutrition research have tolerated this prejudice, young researchers and clinicians today increasingly view this field of research as a 'no-go' area, which will undoubtedly have a negative impact on future healthcare for children. Evidence of this is seen in more recent systematic reviews in which the number of contemporary studies is diminishing, so the review predominantly includes studies published in previous decades, that may or may not be relevant to current policies.

There needs to be a collective understanding of the potential benefits of collaborative and complementary research interests across academic and industry environments. And researchers and clinicians, who are already highly regulated professionals, should be protected and supported in both settings. With a full declaration of interest, they should be encouraged to publish and disseminate their findings at scientific and educational meetings, focusing on the science, and refraining from the promotion of specific commercial products. Rather than create a situation that is high risk for researchers and clinicians, WHO should be working with all stakeholders to establish an academic platform that is creative, multidisciplinary and ethical, and that is underpinned by financial arrangements that ensure all funders are subject to strict standards of governance and regulation.[7]

Sponsorship of educational meetings

In professional and civil society there are few events that do not attract sponsorship. Organizers of events need additional funding, and sponsors are willing to provide financial support. It is recognized that this may be perceived by sponsors as an opportunity to enhance their reputation or benefit commercially, and for these reasons any sponsorship must be subject to strict governance standards. In the National Health Service (NHS) in England, the sponsorship of health-related events by external parties is valued.[4] It is considered that if financial support enables an education and training event to take place, and it benefits healthcare staff and patients, then sponsorship can be justified. Without this funding there might be fewer opportunities for learning, development and partnership-working.

However, it is also recognized that there is potential for conflict of interest between the organizer and the sponsor, particularly regarding the ability to market commercial products or services. As a result, several safeguards are recommended to prevent conflicts occurring.[4,7] These safeguards include the following:

- The event will result in clear benefit to healthcare provision.
- No information will be supplied to the sponsor from which they could gain a commercial advantage.
- The involvement of the sponsor will be clearly identified.
- At the organization's discretion, sponsors or their representatives may attend the event, but cannot influence the content or the main purpose of the event.
- Sponsorship should not equate to endorsement of a company or its products.
- Staff attending should declare their involvement to their organization.

In order for infant-formula companies to provide sponsorship the above conditions should apply, but with a special emphasis on the following aspects:

- The proposed meeting should be limited to scientific and educational matters.
- The sponsor company should not provide input to the content and planning of the meeting.
- There should be equal exposure for all sponsors.

The infant-formula companies have more funding power, so they can buy greater exposure through the current practice of offering platinum, gold and silver sponsorships. This practice should be discontinued: either all sponsors commit to the same funding levels, or there are funding categories that reflect ability to fund, such as private sector, public sector, charity organizations and others.

This is a sensitive area and it will continue to incite emotive views both in favour of sponsorship and against it. It is important for discussions to remain focused on what is best for infants and young children. For example, are the risks of no sponsorship greater than the risks of receiving funding from an infant-formula company? It is recognized that in both developed and developing countries a significant cause of preventable infant and child deaths relates to a failure to provide an appropriate level of clinical expertise and care in the early neonatal period. Therefore the provision of continuing education and training for all clinicians, wherever they are employed, is central to improving infant and child mortality and morbidity. If these training needs can only be provided when sponsorship is available, and if one of the sources of funding is the infant-formula industry, the potential health benefits from the sponsored education need to be balanced against the perceived risks of industry influencing infant feeding. This requires the organizers to adopt the documented standards for sponsorship events, to conduct the process with due diligence, to audit the outcome of the event, and to evaluate the risk with the measured benefits.

To put this issue in a real-world perspective, on current trends fifty-six million children under the age of five are projected to die between 2018 and 2030, with the risk of dying highest in the first month of life. Around 6,700 newborn infants died every day in 2019.[8] As stated by WHO, many of these newborn deaths could be prevented by increasing the level of care during the antenatal period, at the time of birth, and during the postnatal period. To achieve this, health professionals need to receive continuing education and training to develop and maintain their skills. If paediatric and other health organizations take responsibility for organizing educational meetings, and they accept sponsorship under the above conditions, the risks of a material conflict pale into insignificance if the outcome is improved clinical skills that successfully reduces loss of life. In these circumstances, sponsorship can be viewed as a valuable investment in healthcare.

The annual education meeting of the Royal College of Paediatrics and Child Health took place in May 2021. This virtual meeting attracted 1700 attendees from forty-four countries worldwide. The scientific and clinical information from three days of intensive lectures, presentations and discussion was disseminated by the presenters to the attendees and onward to their colleagues in their hospitals, clinics and communities in their respective countries. This sponsored meeting is a highly effective way for paediatricians to receive continuing education and training and ensuring that their profession is qualified to deliver the best care for their child patients worldwide. This should be perceived by WHO as a major contribution to extending coverage of quality care to infants and young children – and not used as another attempt by their officials to unfairly undermine the reputation and commitment of health professionals.

Conflict of interest or interest in conflict?

WHO staff undertook a review of paediatric associations who were receiving sponsorship from infant-formula companies (and other sources). In the subsequently published paper, there were many allegations about the integrity of paediatricians, but no actual evidence of misconduct by any paediatrician was provided.[9]

The paper was published in the *British Medical Journal (Open)*, which also publishes external reviewers' comments. One of the reviewers of their paper stated:

> *"Turning to the discussion, is there any evidence that they (the authors) can draw on, that is specific to these products? Much of what they have is fairly generic, but without knowing the literature in detail, I would have thought that a call to [the Policy Director] at Baby Milk Action would provide any material that exists. If, for example, they could illustrate the discussion with some of the case studies that have been published on, for example, the tobacco and soft drinks industries it would greatly strengthen their case for action".*

The follow-up response from the authors was:

> *"We have added an example that was published in British Medical Journal last year about a dramatic rise in prescriptions for specialized formula for cow's-milk protein allergy. There appear to have been significant conflicts of interest on the expert panels that have published guidelines on the topic".*[9]

Having been prompted by the reviewer, who clearly had his own views on this matter, the authors included the following paragraph in their final version of the paper:

> *"For example, van Tulleken has noted that prescriptions of specialist formula milks for cow's-milk protein allergy have increased dramatically over the past decade based on the guidelines of several expert groups.[9] Ten of the twelve authors of the 2012 European Society for Paediatric Gastroenterology, Hepatology, and Nutrition guidelines on diagnosis and management of cow's-milk protein allergy and all authors of the international Milk Allergy in Primary Care (iMAP) guideline on cow's milk allergy declared financial interests with infant formula manufacturers".*

It appears from this article that WHO have now ventured into investigative journalism. Is this really the role of WHO officials and is this opinion or evidence?

It is necessary to reflect on the previous paper by van Tulleken, which was published in the *BMJ* and is a most unusual contribution to an international scientific journal.[10] The author (just one) is an honorary senior lecturer at University College London and is very active as a medical journalist and television presenter. The content of the paper was predominantly based on telephone conversations with a range of people, including three representatives from WHO, one of whom is the lead author of the *BMJ Open* article. All three were co-authors of the *Lancet* letter from WHO regarding paediatricians. It is noted that van Tulleken's paper was commissioned by the *BMJ*, but the arrangements relating to the commissioning process were not published (although it can be assumed that the Editor of the *BMJ* was familiar with his views). Interestingly, it appears that the *BMJ* staff undertook most of the telephone conversations and information gathering. Here are some examples.

> *"The [BMJ] has confirmed that materials produced by formula manufacturers were displayed and distributed at events at St Thomas."*

> *"Clinicians and patients who spoke to the [BMJ] are concerned at the wide availability of industry funded online information."*

> *"The [BMJ] attempted to contact all the authors of these guidelines and received six replies from authors with declared conflicts of interest."*

Van Tulleken's declaration of interest was:

> *"I have read and understood [BMJ] policy on declaration of interests and have no relevant interests to declare."*

This is despite evidence of collaboration between the author and *BMJ* staff, who are not acknowledged as co-authors.

The rise in the profile of cow's milk allergy and the need for cow's-milk protein-free formulas is interpreted by WHO as a consequence of researchers being influenced by financial incentives from industry, which has led to overdiagnosis and increased purchase of cow's-milk protein-free formulas. These are serious allegations, and it is irresponsible to make these claims without robust evidence.

An alternative and more rational explanation for the rise in the prevalence of cow's milk allergy is that it was previously under-diagnosed, and it is a consequence of the research by scientists and clinicians that this condition is now more widely recognized and is actively investigated.

Note that by establishing the diagnosis with a low-cost elimination diet and introducing a cow's-milk protein-free formula, the diagnosis and treatment can be established without the need for expensive diagnostic tests or medicines, and therefore the current recommended management of this condition is extremely cost-effective.

The abstract of the ESPGHAN guideline on the diagnosis and management of cow's-milk protein allergy in infants and children is presented in Box 15.1 (*overpage*). It provides clear evidence of a rational approach to a clinical condition that can cause significant symptoms in early childhood, which (in exceptional cases) can be life threatening. The guideline guards against excessive investigation and unnecessarily prolonged elimination diets, and it also makes reference to avoidable healthcare costs. It is difficult to see how this can be interpreted as 'bad practice' and why this has provoked WHO to make their unfortunate remarks. It appears that WHO and their colleagues in breastfeeding activist groups are prepared to take any action that may inflict reputational damage on healthcare professionals who have collaborated in any way with industry.

In response to the WHO paper in *BMJ Open*, a position paper was published in the journal *Frontiers in Pediatrics*. It was co-authored by representatives from seven European paediatric associations.[11]

- European Academy of Paediatrics (EAP)
- European Society for Paediatric Gastroenterology, Hepatology and Nutrition (ESPGHAN)
- European Society for Paediatric Infectious Diseases (ESPID)
- European Society of Paediatric and Neonatal Intensive Care (ESPNIC)
- European Society for Paediatric Nephrology (ESPN)
- European Society for Paediatric Research (ESPR)
- European Society of Emergency Medicine (EUSEM) paediatric section.

Box 15.1: Diagnostic approach and management of cow's-milk protein allergy in infants and children from ESPGHAN GI Committee Practical Guidelines—Abstract (2012).

Source: https://journals.lww.com/jpgn/Fulltext/2012/08000/Diagnostic_Approach_and_Management_of_Cow_s_Milk.28.aspx/.

- **Objectives:** This guideline provides recommendations for the diagnosis and management of suspected cow's-milk protein allergy (CMPA) in Europe. It presents a practical approach with a diagnostic algorithm and is based on recently published evidence-based guidelines on CMPA.

- **Diagnosis:** If CMPA is suspected by history and examination, then strict allergen avoidance is initiated. In certain circumstances (e.g. a clear history of immediate symptoms, a life-threatening reaction with a positive test for CMP-specific IgE), the diagnosis can be made without a milk challenge. In all other circumstances, a controlled oral food challenge (open or blind) under medical supervision is required to confirm or exclude the diagnosis of CMPA.

- **Treatment:** In breastfed infants, the mother should start a strict CMP-free diet. Non-breastfed infants with confirmed CMPA should receive an extensively hydrolyzed protein-based formula with proven efficacy in appropriate clinical trials; amino acids–based formulae are reserved for certain situations. Soy protein formula, if tolerated, is an option beyond 6 months of age. Nutritional counselling and regular monitoring of growth are mandatory in all age groups requiring CMP exclusion.

- **Re-evaluation:** Patients should be re-evaluated every 6 to 12 months to assess whether they have developed tolerance to CMP. This is achieved in >75% by 3 years of age and >90% by 6 years of age. Inappropriate or overly long dietary eliminations should be avoided. Such restrictions may impair the quality of life of both child and family, induce improper growth, and incur unnecessary health care costs.

These organizations confirmed their support for WHO recommendations on infant feeding, but they made several points relating to relations between paediatric associations and infant-formula industry with specific reference to funding educational meetings, as quoted here:

"Families need counselling on infant-feeding choices by informed paediatricians and other healthcare professionals who have access to current evidence."

"Paediatricians and other healthcare professionals can obtain current information through congresses and other forms of continuing medical education that should be directed and supervised by independent paediatric organizations or public bodies."

"In order to avoid bias due to conflict of interest, commercial enterprises should not direct and offer scientific events and continuing medical education for healthcare professionals."

"However, financial support from commercial enterprises for congresses, continuing medical education activities and other activities of learned societies and professional organizations is an acceptable option if agreed scientific, ethical,

societal and legal standards are followed, which includes ensuring no influence of commercial enterprises on the program, content of activities and transparency on financial support.

"Public–private research collaborations for improving and evaluating pharmaceuticals, vaccines, medical devices, dietetic products and other products and services for children are encouraged, provided they are guided by the goal of enhancing child health and are performed following current ethical, scientific and societal standards.

"Investment of public funding for research aiming at promoting child health, as well as for continuing medical education, should be strengthened."

While the paediatric associations enthusiastically support breastfeeding, they also recognize that healthy infants that are not (or not fully) breastfed require a breastmilk substitute, and that many sick infants require therapeutic dietetic products. Both of these should be of the highest achievable quality to support child health and wellbeing. The paediatric associations strongly disagreed with the view expressed by WHO in the *BMJ Open* article that such products would generally be *"goods that are not in the best interest of child health"*. They emphasized that infant formulas are needed for infants who are not breastfed for different reasons to support their health as best as possible. Infant formulas or supplements to breastfeeding can even be an essential medical requirement for some infants, for example those that are born very preterm, or with inherited metabolic disorders, intestinal failure, complex food allergies, congenital cardiac lesions, enterocolitic syndromes, severe gastroesophageal reflux and neurodisability.

The position paper enforces the point that paediatricians and other healthcare professionals are fully aware that providers of pharmaceuticals and vaccines, medical devices, dietetic products and other products and services have commercial interests, but they are able to critically evaluate the communications they have and make decisions that are in the best interest of their patients.

Moreover, if WHO or any other organization or individuals have concerns regarding their probity, scientists and clinicians are subject to professional regulatory standards and can be referred to a relevant regulatory authority for investigation. In the meantime, without providing any proven lawful evidence of guilt, policy-makers should resist attempting to undermine the reputation of researchers and clinicians with evidence that is no more than personal opinion or prejudice.

As noted in the European paediatric associations' repost, there are many other examples of highly effective collaboration between researchers, clinicians and the infant-formula industry that have led to the development of specialized formulas. A stellar example of this is the early diagnosis of phenylketonuria (PKU) and the availability of phenylalanine-free infant formulas which, over the last fifty years, have changed the outcome of this condition from severe brain damage and early death to someone leading a normal healthy life.[12]

Therefore, rather than 'disentangling' researchers and clinicians from the infant-formula industry, there should be a greater focus on how these collaborations can further improve all aspects of infant and young-child nutrition, with the relationship being subject to independent governance and regulation. In my opinion WHO's current campaign to discredit the scientists and clinicians involved in this clinical area, by casting aspersions that they are servants of the infant-formula industry (and doing so without offering any proper evidence) is a sad reflection on an organization that should be a beacon of integrity and professionalism.

The interface between policy-makers, paediatricians and industry

The alleged conflicts of interest within the infant-feeding community highlight different viewpoints on how industry is perceived by policy-makers and healthcare professionals. This reflects their different roles and objectives, whereby policy-makers have responsibility for the development of policy for populations (nationally or globally), whereas health professionals are focused on providing care for individual children and their families. Policymakers, especially WHO, tend to develop one-size-fits-all global infant-feeding policies, in contrast with the more grounded healthcare approach in which the needs of children are met by providing individualized clinical care.

Of course, clinical practice is not an exact science (some maintain it is an art), with the underlying assertion that the best clinicians are not only knowledgeable and experienced but also have reliable clinical judgment.[13] Good judgement is extremely important in managing infant-feeding issues, as there are many nutritional and non-nutritional confounding factors, including health status, growth and development, and culture and socio-economic circumstances, that need to be taken into consideration when developing infant-feeding policy and practice. With these different approaches it is not surprising that health practitioners can find themselves making some clinical decisions that they believe are in the best interests of the child, but may not be compatible with global policies, including the Code. A greater understanding of these specific circumstances may reduce the levels of acrimony generated by claims of conflict of interest or non-compliance with the Code.

The argument that clinicians who collaborate with industry have potential conflicts of interest is being strenuously pursued by the Editor of the *BMJ* who has made a decision not to accept clinical editorials and education articles from authors that have had "*relevant financial or other ties with industry*".[14] This presumably excludes scientists involved in the development of a vaccine against Ebola or Coronavirus who, during this critically important development, held a contract with a pharmaceutical company. In this scenario, what is the conflict of interest? And how great is the risk?

The alleged conflict of interest is that the scientists will have been unduly influenced by the drug company and therefore cannot be trusted to provide an independent opinion on matters relating to their experience of vaccine development. Is this risk greater than any risks that might be associated with preventing readers from learning about the scientist's contribution to vaccine development? Are the actions being taken by the journal professionally and ethically acceptable?

The most recent experience relating to Covid-19 is that many scientists from academia and industry, who have had professional, financial and other "*ties*" with industry, have been communicating their experience in many formats and this has been of considerable interest to scientific colleagues, the wider media and the populations, many of whom remain "*at risk*" from this infection (see the correspondence in the *Addendum* to this chapter).

Both WHO and breastfeeding activist groups have stated that collaboration of health professionals with industry on research or educational matters, particularly if there is associated industry funding, is contrary to what is recommended in the Code, and that health professionals have a conflict of interest.

As described previously, the issue of conflict of interest tends to focus on whether the conflict relates to financial interests, and there are examples of WHO making claims of conflict of interest against researchers and clinicians who have contributed to the scientific literature on infant feeding – and correctly declared that they have received funding for research or honoraria for lectures. WHO's claims are most often made when WHO are not in agreement with the data and outcomes that have been reported. It is important to note that *insinuation* of conflict of interest, that is not substantiated by formal evidence of criminality or professional misconduct, is unacceptable. And it raises questions about the integrity of those who are making the allegations.

Recognizing that a conflict of interest can be related to non-financial issues, decisions on global policy have undoubtedly been made by some stakeholders who take a longstanding negative stance against the infant-formula industry. This has been manifested by failure to engage with industry, by preventing collaboration between industry and other stakeholders, and by providing support for boycotts, legal action and sanctions against industry. Interestingly, they do not declare these material conflicts of interest.

Even with the best partnership-working, some claims of conflict of interest will inevitably emerge, but it is important that any claims of conflict are responsible and proportionate. For this to be achieved there must be a system for clearly determining the level of material conflict that may influence judgement on health-related matters, and thus present as a real conflict of interest. This requires a careful balance of the benefits against the risks, with a process that demonstrates due diligence and ensures that the evaluation does not fall victim to further conflicts of interest. A blatant conflict of interest should be easily identified, however assessment of a *potential* conflict of interest introduces elements of judgement and opinion, rather than *fact*. In these circumstances, there may be a fine dividing line between good judgement, self-interest and conflict of interest. Given the potential level of uncertainty, it is particularly important that conflict of interest is not used as a tool by individuals or organizations to advance self-interest and create further division and distrust.

WHO, with support from breastfeeding interest groups, frequently claim examples of conflict of interest committed by other organizations within the infant-feeding community. In their letter to *The Lancet*, the WHO officials stated that paediatricians:

"… need to adopt codes of conduct and practices that protect their vested interests".[3]

It must be understood that paediatricians' vested interests are the health and wellbeing of their patients, and the fundamental issue is that each of the stakeholders have a different perspective on 'vested interest'. This is most evident in the establishment of the NetCode monitoring system set up by WHO.

NetCode was formed through a partnership between WHO, UN system organizations, WHO collaborating centres, NGOs that are particularly active in supporting breastfeeding and selected WHO and UN member states.[15] Their key objective is to monitor compliance with the Code and to:

"… hold manufacturers, distributors, retail outlets, the healthcare system and healthcare workers to account for their breaches of national laws and/or the Code".

When violations are detected, they encourage governments to impose sanctions as permitted by national legislation. However, the organizations that initiated this process, and also participate as monitors, have a long history of preventing industry involvement in all aspects of infant-feeding policy and practice. Thus they themselves have a material conflict of interest.

NetCode is clearly divisive, with one half of the infant-feeding community monitoring the other half – there is not a reciprocal arrangement. No reference is made to parents. Therefore, which side of the divide they would cast their allegiance is uncertain. Moreover, NetCode is clearly not an independent judiciary process. Further to this, with the concerns expressed about sponsorship, NetCode is not publicly funded and is currently sponsored by the Bill & Melinda Gates Foundation.

Is there a way forward?

It is evident that infant-feeding research, development and practice is becoming caught in an expanding web of conflicts of interest, and therefore a rational way forward needs to be considered.

In 2015, WHO convened a technical consultation on 'Addressing and managing conflicts of interest in the planning and delivery of nutrition programmes at country level'.[16-20] It was indicated that the consultation on this complex issue was the beginning of a process that aimed to develop risk assessment, disclosure and management tools for safeguarding member states against conflicts of interest in nutrition programmes. The working document for the technical consultation included three definitions of conflict of interest,[16] the first being:

> *"An actual conflict of interest arises when a vested interest has the potential to unduly influence official or agency judgement/action through the monetary or material benefits it confers on the official or agency".*

The second definition was:

> *"The perceived conflict of interest that arises when a vested interest has the potential to unduly influence official or agency judgement/action through the non-monetary or non-material influences it exerts on the official or agency".*

And the third:

> *"An outcome-based conflict of interest arises when a vested interest, involved in the policymaking or policy-implementation process, seeks outcomes that are*

inconsistent with the demonstrable public interest. This applies to issues where there is consensus on the public interest and where a particular interest, by the nature of its mission, pursues goals that are in contradiction with that interest".

It is noted that the participants in the Technical Consultation included twenty members from WHO and twenty-five external members, predominantly academics and public health officials. There was no representation from the food industry. It is clearly important that if the outcome of these discussions is going to achieve an acceptable level of compliance, key stakeholder representation would be advisable at the outset. Exclusion at the planning stage is the forerunner of resistance at the implementation stage, and this became evident at the subsequent on-line consultation phase of this process.

Invitations were sent to a wide range of centres of academia, public health, non-governmental organizations, and the private sector, including food and beverage, and to all Member States with a copy of a draft *Approach For The Prevention And Management Of Conflicts Of Interest*, which included a six-step protocol.[17] Probably the most significant finding from the consultation was that only six countries responded, three were from high-income and three from upper-middle income countries, with no responses from lower or lower-middle income countries. It is important to reflect on why this topic, which is considered to be of high priority for organizations who take issue with the behaviour and attitude of the food industry, did not generate national government interest.

Allowing for the limited response to the consultation, three conceptualizations of conflict of interest emerged.[18-19] First, was a concept of collaboration and partnership, with the matter being viewed as effectively addressed by requirements for individual disclosure and there was a concern that more invasive restrictions would inhibit partnership approaches. This concept received most support from private sector respondents. Second, was a concept of conflict and restricted engagement and need for effective management of food industry interests and public health goals. This received support from the majority of civil society organizations and four of the member states (Brazil, Canada, Columbia, Namibia). Third, was a concept where there was a fundamental rejection of the legitimacy or efficacy of any multistakeholder and partnership governance models in relation to food policy and this was supported by a small mixed group of five respondents, including IBFAN who was probably the most strident.

From the process so far, it is evident that achieving agreement on a single global policy on conflict of interest that addresses issues of planning and delivery of nutrition programmes at country level, is going to be difficult. An academic review conducted in 2021, on the proposed WHO tool to support member states in preventing and managing conflict of interest in nutrition policy concluded that:

> *"Submissions on the WHO tool illustrate how contrasting positions on conflict of interest are central to understanding broader debates in nutrition policy and across global health governance.[20] Effective health governance requires greater understanding of how conflict of interest can be conceptualised and managed amid high levels of contestation on policy engagement with commercial sector actors. This requires both ongoing innovation in governance tools and more extensive conceptual and empirical research".*

Moreover, in the on-line feedback, the Cochrane Collaboration commented that there is no disclosure of conflicts of interest for those who were involved in drafting the papers and they also noted that there was no description of who should conduct the risk assessments and they specifically emphasised the need for Member States to have a committee with relevant knowledge of the nutrition field to be convened, and that the committee members be free of conflicts of interest. This view is relevant to the discussion on claims of conflicts of interest by WHO officials against stakeholders who are perceived not to be complying with WHO recommendations. It is evident in these circumstances that WHO is not free of conflicts of interest, therefore clarity on the role of WHO in relation to conflict of interest may be a helpful starting point for addressing the wider issues of conflict of interest within infant-feeding policy and practice.

Should WHO disentangle itself from conflict of interest?

In relation to infant feeding, the dominant influence on policy and practice is the decision-making process at the WHO/WHA level and this is significantly influenced by a key objective of WHO, which is to promote breastfeeding as a global necessity and dissuade parents from using infant formula. However this binary approach does not necessarily fit with the many variables associated with infant-feeding practice. Consequently, progress and compliance have been challenging, and WHO has attempted to strengthen the message by taking actions that trend towards conflict of interest. For example, there is clear evidence of discrimination against individuals and organizations that have 'ties' with the infant-formula industry, the nature of which may vary considerably but decisions on non-selection for policy development appear to be absolute. This contrasts with the benevolence towards breastfeeding organizations that are welcomed; this is most evident with WHO and UNICEF's involvement in the institution and coordination of the Global Breastfeeding Collective that enables these organizations to have direct contact with the WHO officials who are setting policy.

The vested interest of WHO officials and activists for breastfeeding may ideologically be correct but, as indicated in the above definitions, it is important to consider whether their vested interest has:

> "… the potential to unduly influence official or agency judgement/action through the non-monetary or non-material influences it exerts on the official or agency, or whether it has a "consensus of the public interest", and whether the vested interest "pursues goals that are in contradiction with that interest?".

With WHO being the policymaker and the decision maker in relation to infant feeding, it is important to have clarity around the different roles of the WHO officials, to ensure that there is a clear understanding between what is official WHO business and communication, and what may be perceived as communications from WHO officials that are more personal and represent self-interest when a declaration at the end of a paper or letter they have written states that the content "*does not necessarily represent the views, decisions, or policies of WHO*". This statement, which is used frequently by WHO officials, raises the question as to whether information from WHO officials should be exclusively considered as the views and opinions of the WHO? Or can WHO officials use their professional position in the WHO to exercise their personal views on infant feeding in order to influence stakeholders, journal editors and activists?

For example, the WHO officials who wrote to *The Lancet* regarding the Royal College of Paediatrics and Child Health and were critical of the role played by paediatricians in the use of sponsorship. They provided a declaration that said:

> "*The authors alone are responsible for the views expressed in this letter and they do not necessarily represent the views, decisions, or policies of WHO. We declare no competing interests*".

As previously indicated, in this declaration the authors have failed to indicate *which* views in the letter are directly related to WHO policy and *which* are the opinions of the authors. And despite this uncertainty, they declare that they have "*no competing interests*".

With reference to the definitions and scenarios above, it could be concluded that the objective of their intervention was to use their WHO position to influence the readers of *The Lancet* of their perception of the RCPCH behaving inappropriately, and also to draw attention to WHA resolutions with which they will have been closely involved. This does appear to be a 'vested interest' *and* a potential conflict of interest. So what is the status of this letter? Is it an official communication between WHO and the RCPCH? Or is it an example of WHO officials doing a spot of freelancing and using their WHO positions to give some credibility to their views? Is their motive to encourage support for the WHO Code and resolutions – or is it an opportunity to undermine the influence and authority of the RCPCH? Overall, is this acceptable practice? And would it not be more appropriate for the WHO to approach the RCPCH directly in an official capacity, which would be more in-keeping with standard governance procedures?

The WHO officials who were involved in the *BMJ Open* paper, which also challenged the use of sponsorship from infant-formula companies, declared:

> "*Funding: All authors are staff or interns at the World Health Organization. No separate funding was obtained for this study. Disclaimer: The authors alone are responsible for the views expressed in this article and they do not necessarily represent the decisions, policy or views of the institutions with which they are affiliated. Competing interests: None declared*".

In this declaration it is evident that this paper is not an official WHO document because it states:

> "*The authors alone are responsible for the views expressed in this article and they do not necessarily represent the decisions, policy or views of the institutions with which they are affiliated*".

So once again, it is difficult to be clear where accountability lies, but the authors appear to be channelling their personal views from their positions within WHO to the *BMJ Open* journal. It is difficult to understand *how* they do not have competing interests as they are employees of WHO, and some are actively involved in infant-feeding policy. The comment that "*No separate funding was obtained for this study*" indicates that it was funded by core WHO funds provided by national governments, and this again raises questions about the status of this paper.

It appears to be an example of freelancing by WHO employees – but funded by WHO – and clarity regarding the validity of their roles is required. Moreover, as already discussed, there is some discomfort regarding the quality and integrity of the paper. The WHO official defending the re-defining of breastmilk substitutes, whereby all milk products marketed for children up to the age of three years are understood to be breastmilk substitutes, declared that:

> *"The author is a staff member of the World Health Organization. The author alone is responsible for the views expressed in this commentary and they do not necessarily represent the decisions, policy or views of the World Health Organization".*

Why not? It is the WHA that has "welcomed" this recommendation, which will impact on most families worldwide, and therefore it is the views and explanations of the WHO and WHA that health professionals and the general public wish to hear?

The author also declared there were *"no conflicts of interest to report"*. Relating this declaration to the fact that the WHO official was a member of STAG, and closely involved in the development of that specific WHO policy recommendation that has significantly changed the definition of a breastmilk substitute, it is difficult to comprehend the *"no conflicts of interest"* claim. Furthermore, this change has had a major impact on families – therefore this *does* appear to be a vested interest, one that has:

> *"... influenced the policymaking or policy-implementation process and sought outcomes that are inconsistent with the demonstrable public interest".*

With the aforementioned controversy surrounding this recommendation, an official WHO statement would have been expected.

Conclusion

Much of the acrimony, division and conflict surrounding infant-feeding policy relate to interpretation of WHO's recommendations and the need for relevance to contemporary life, but WHO has chosen to stand firm on their twenty- to forty-year-old policies and move to protect them from challenge by responding with claims of conflict of interest as noted above.

As WHO has a vested interest in these policies, WHO should not be adjudicating on conflict of interest; perhaps WHO needs to remain neutral on the potential issues of conflict of interest and allow an independent organization to assess and cast judgement. Additionally, if policies are not undergoing regular reviews and updates, especially over periods of decades, then the relevance of these policies will continue to be challenged, and eventually standard governance procedures will need to prevail.

The foundations of good practice depend on all organizations involved in the infant-feeding community being able to demonstrate acceptable standards for professionalism, governance and regulation, which should be assessed by an independent regulatory body. Organizations that are considered by the regulatory body to not be meeting these standards should not participate in infant-feeding policy-making. Conflict of interest should be monitored and addressed (if proven), but there is evidence that claims of conflict of interest are embedded in underlying issues of acrimony and mistrust.

Systemic changes are therefore required, including the establishment of an environment in which all partners collaborate to develop a mutual understanding of the principles of infant-feeding policy and practice. This should include an acknowledgement that self-interest, which at times may be perceived as a conflict, needs to be managed effectively, that progress can be achieved by appropriate compromise and incremental change, and that the overall objective is to support and protect infants and their families.

Addendum

This chapter is based on a previously published article: Forsyth S (2019) Infant feeding and conflict of interest: a healthcare perspective. *Annals of Nutrition and Metabolism* 75, 252–55. DOI: 10.1159/000504775. Other related correspondence is: Forsyth S (2015) The *British Medical Journal* should not take the law into its own hands on competing interests, *British Medical Journal* 350, g7766 (see *https://DOI.org/10.1136/bmj.g7766/*). This letter is reproduced in Box 15.2.

Box 15.2: Letter to the *British Medical Journal* (2015)

The case for discriminating against clinicians whose professional interest leads them to collaborate with industry needs to be built on evidence rather than perception.[a] Reference is made to two papers, both of which are low-response questionnaires for doctors, requesting their perception of the validity and believability on hypothetical papers that made no declaration of interest, were grant funded, or were funded by a company with which the lead author was financially involved. Not surprisingly, these study designs came up with the answer that believability ratings were lowest for the industry funded paper.[b,c]

Research misconduct can occur at all levels, from an individual researcher to the department or institution, journals and the funding bodies.[d] Bias in educational articles can reflect many factors, including associations with research funding organizations, government bodies and industry, or simply being employed by a university with a policy of 'publish or perish'. Rather than take 'the law into its own hands' the BMJ should reinforce current conditions of publication, including a full declaration of all potential conflicts of interest; editorial teams and peer reviewers of journal submissions should carefully assess the scientific content and validity of all papers, including editorials and educational articles. Readers should then be allowed to make their own judgement about the article's value to them. All contributors to medical journals need to adhere to professional standards, including probity, and if there is evidence that standards are breached, referral to our professional bodies or law masters should be the way forward.

Sources cited in the letter

[a] Chew M, Brizzell C, Abbasi K, Godlee F (2014) Medical journals and industry ties. *British Medical Journal* 349, g7197.

[b] Schroter S, Morris J, Chaudhry S, Smith, R, Barratt H (2004) Does the type of competing interest affect readers' perceptions of the credibility of research? Randomised trial. *British Medical Journal 328, 742.*

[c] Kesselheim AS, Robertson CT, Myers JA, *et al.* (2012) A randomized study of how physicians interpret research funding disclosures. *New England Journal of Medicine* 367, 1119–27.

[d] Sarwar U, Nicolaou M (2012) Fraud and deceit in medical research. *Journal of Research in Medical Science* 17, 1077–81.

References

1. Forsyth JS (2010) *International Code of Marketing of Breastmilk Substitutes* – three decades later time for hostilities to be replaced by effective national and international governance. *Archives of Diseases in Childhood* 95, 769–70.

2. WHO (1981) *International Code of Marketing of Breastmilk Substitutes.* Available at: https://apps.who.int/iris/bitstream/handle/10665/40382/9241541601.pdf?sequence=1&isAllowed=y (last accessed August 2022).

3. Costello A, Branca F, Rollins N, *et al.* (2017) Health professional associations and industry funding. *The Lancet* 389, 597–98.

4. NHS England (2017) *Managing conflicts of interest in the NHS. Guidance for staff and organizations.* Available at: https://www.england.nhs.uk/wp–content/uploads/2017/02/guidance–managing–conflicts–of–interest–nhs.pdf/ (last accessed August 2022).

5. Godlee F (2018) Disentangling ourselves from 'Big Formula'. *British Medical Journal* 363, k5146.

6. Forsyth S (2018) Should the World Health Organization relax its policy of non-cooperation with the infant food industry? *Annals of Nutrition and Metabolism* 73, 160–62.

7. Forsyth S (2019) Infant feeding and conflict of interest: a healthcare perspective. *Annals of Nutrition and Metabolism.* DOI 10.1159/000504775.

8. UN (2018) *Levels and trends in child mortality report 2018.* Available at: https://www.un.org/en/development/desa/population/publications/mortality/child–mortality–report–2018.asp/ (last accessed August 2022).

9. Grummer-Strawn LM, Holliday F, Jungo KT, Rollins N (2019) Sponsorship of national and regional professional paediatrics associations by companies that make breastmilk substitutes: evidence from a review of official websites. *BMJ Open* 9, e029035.

10. Van Tulleken C (2018) Overdiagnosis and industry influence: how cow's-milk protein allergy is extending the reach of infant formula manufacturers. *British Medical Journal* 363, k5056.

11. Bognar Z, De Luca D, Domellöf M, *et al.* (2020) Promoting breastfeeding and interaction of pediatric associations with providers of nutritional products. *Frontiers in Pediatrics* 8, 562870. DOI: 10.3389/fped.2020.562870.

12. Pinto A, Adams S, Ahring K, *et al.* (2018) Early feeding practices in infants with phenylketonuria across Europe. *Molecular Genetics and Metabolism Reports* 16, 82 89.

13. Panda SC (2006) Medicine: science or art? *Mens Sana Monographs* 4, 127–38.

14. Godlee F (2014) Medical journals and industry ties. *British Medical Journal* 349, g7197.

15. WHO/UN Children's Fund (2017) *NetCode toolkit. Monitoring the marketing of breastmilk substitutes: protocol for ongoing monitoring systems.* Licence CC BY-NC-SA 3.0 IGO. Available at: https://apps.who.int/iris/bitstream/handle/10665/259441/9789241513180-eng.pdf (last accessed September 2022).

16. WHO (2017) *Safeguarding against possible conflicts of interest in nutrition programmes.* Available at: http://apps.who.int/gb/ebwha/pdf_files/EB142/B142_23–en.pdf?ua=1 (last accessed September 2022),

17. WHO. *Addressing and managing conflicts of interest in the planning and delivery of nutrition programmes at country level. Report of a technical consultation convened in Geneva, Switzerland* (8–9 October 2015). Available at: https://apps.who.int/iris/bitstream/handle/10665/206554/9789241510530_eng.pdf?sequence=1&isAllowed=y (last accessed August 2022).

18. WHO (2017) *Approach for the prevention and management of conflicts of interest in the policy development and implementation of nutrition programmes at country level Feedback on the WHO consultation.* Available at: https://www.who.int/news-room/events/detail/2017/09/11/default-calendar/safeguarding-against-possible-conflicts-of-interest-in-nutrition-programmes-consultation-comments (last accessed August 2022).

19. WHO (2017) *Safeguarding against possible conflicts of interest in nutrition programmes. Draft approach for the prevention and management of conflicts of interest in the policy development and implementation of nutrition programmes at country level. Report by the Director-General. 4 December 2017.* Available at: https://apps.who.int/iris/bitstream/handle/10665/274165/B142_23-en.pdf?sequence=1&isAllowed=y (last accessed August 2022).

20. Ralston R, Hill SE, da Silva Gomes F, Collin J. Towards preventing and managing conflict of interest in nutrition policy? An analysis of submissions to a consultation on a draft WHO tool. *International Journal of Health Policy Management* 2021, 10(5), 255–65.

CHAPTER 16

An independent review of infant-feeding policy-making is long overdue

As has been emphasized in this critique, partnership-working – especially between WHO and the infant-food industry – has been tainted by its history of dissension, and as a result infant-feeding issues relating to policy and practice that were prominent four decades ago remain unresolved.[1]

Stakeholder conflict in the context of disappointing global breastfeeding rates, deficiencies in complementary feeding, the double burden of childhood malnutrition and poor progress in achieving sustainable developmental goals certainly justifies an independent review of the strengths and limitations of the current policy-making process. The failure of WHO/WHA to initiate an independent review during the last forty years is indeed surprising and reflects a serious lack of governance of a system that is responsible for the most vulnerable populations worldwide. Key objectives could be to determine:

- how an 'enabling' environment can be achieved across infant-feeding partnerships
- how the diverse nutritional requirements of infants and young children worldwide can be effectively delivered
- how policies can be designed to mitigate against future crises in childhood nutrition.

Within this remit, there are several key determinants that could form the substance of the review. They are précised in this chapter.

Roles and responsibilities of WHO, WHA and governments

The constitution of WHO states that their role is to act as the directing and coordinating authority on international health, and to assist governments – upon request – in strengthening a range of health services, including maternal and child health. The constitution also states that national governments have responsibility for the health of their citizens, which can only be fulfilled by the provision of adequate health and social measures. For the global and national approach to be effective there has to be clarity on their roles and responsibilities within strategic and operational global and national parameters.

In WHO's global infant and young-child feeding strategy, which was endorsed by the WHA in 2002 and published in 2003, the recommendations range from general principles on direction and support to specific operational details, including the number of months every woman worldwide should breastfeed. Their Code is a highly operational document that provides detailed instruction to industry, health professionals, health systems and the general public, but there are no similar recommendations for WHO or WHA or breastfeeding advocacy and activist groups.

The WHO infant-feeding strategy states that each partner should acknowledge and embrace its responsibilities for improving the feeding of infants and young children, and that all partners should work together to fully achieve the strategy's aim and objectives. However, in a recently published comprehensive, independent assessment of the Code,[2] it is stated that:

> "... the entire space surrounding the Code remains entrenched with hostility between industry and NGO institutions, many of whom are barely on open speaking terms with one another".

The Code has not been updated since it was published in 1981. The WHA has chosen to publish *ad hoc* resolutions following their meetings, and these 'subsequent resolutions' are embedded in WHO and WHA literature. With the brevity of the resolution documents, policy statements may only be recorded within WHO's secretariat working documents.[3] However, this process lacks transparency. As a minimum, it has been suggested, WHO and WHA should take steps to present the Code and subsequent resolutions as a coherent set of standards.[2]

Transformational change should ensure that the roles and responsibilities of WHO, WHA and governments are distinct and complementary, and that global and national recommendations are optimally balanced to ensure that parents receive recommendations that are most pertinent to their children. With a global background of extensive diversity, some WHO recommendations (including the most recent statement that all milk products marketed for children up to the age of three years should be considered as breastmilk substitutes)[4] can be perceived by parents as lacking sensitivity and credibility. As a consequence, parental non-compliance remains high. Many of them choose to develop a personal infant feeding plan that they believe will best serve their own infants' needs. To address this issue, governments should embrace the underlying principles of WHO and WHA but be expected to take responsibility for the development of national recommendations on infant feeding – recommendations that more closely reflect national needs and are supported by national stakeholders.

Roles and responsibilities of policy-makers, health professionals and industry

In response to the unethical marketing and promotion of infant formulas by industry during the 1960s and 1970s, the WHA endorsed the Code in 1981. However, because of continuing violations, the WHA continues to issue resolutions that add further restrictions to the activities of industry. In addition, many of the breastfeeding advocacy and activist groups have continued to support protests, boycotts and legal actions against infant-formula companies, especially Nestlé. Despite four decades of anti-industry activity, however, non-compliance with WHO infant-feeding recommendations persists. Nestlé is now the largest food and beverage company in the world. Formula sales are rising, and nutrition-related factors contribute to 45% of deaths in children under five years of age.

The leading global health and nutrition institutions have adopted positions of non-cooperation with industry when all stakeholders should be collectively focusing on the development of child-feeding policies that reflect diverse nutritional and socioeconomic circumstances. This approach is professionally and ethically wrong. Moreover, collateral damage is now impacting on all stakeholders, including scientists, health practitioners and families.

Understanding the interface between policy-makers, health professionals and industry is critically important if multi-professional delivery of effective infant-feeding policy is going to be successful. Policy-makers have responsibility for developing policy for populations that may be national or global, but the one-size-fits-all global infant-feeding policies recommended by WHO are in contrast to a healthcare approach that is focused on providing care for individual children and their families.

Clinical practice is not an exact science and good judgement is extremely important for managing infant-feeding issues as there are so many nutritional and non-nutritional confounding factors that need to be considered. Because of these different approaches it is not surprising that health practitioners find themselves making some clinical decisions that they believe are in the best interests of the child, but may not be compliant with global policies, including the Code.

If health professionals are to provide the best nutritional care for the children in their care, there will be circumstances in which good practice will be to consult with industry, and this may lead to collaborative research. It is therefore essential to foster an enabling environment across infant-feeding partnerships that will ensure the best nutrition can be developed and delivered to all infants and young children, especially those living in the most difficult circumstances.

Effective leadership is clearly critical if a unifying approach to the delivery of the best policies and practices is to be achieved, and current leadership actions and behaviours need to be closely examined.

Parent-friendly policies

A review of public engagement and policy-making stated that effective policy requires transparency, accessibility to and responsiveness of as wide a range of citizens as possible.[5] These elements must be applied at all stages of the design and delivery of public services in order to be successful, as this will promote better understanding of the evolving and diverse needs within populations. Furthermore, it is important to reach out beyond the 'usual suspects' and avoid the risk of 'policy hijacking' by the vociferous few who are unlikely to be representative of the silent majority.

As I have said before, compliance with infant-feeding policy requires consensus from parents, and consensus from parents requires consultation with parents. The needs of a population evolve, and all policies have to adapt to societal change. This is exemplified by the rapid expansion of the female workforce and laws on freedom of information, which underlines the importance of information access, not only as a human right but also as a right to ensure good governance.

The Code states that parents can *only* receive scientific and factual information from healthcare workers. However, today's public expect to have immediate access to electronically delivered information and can commonly access search engines, assimilate information and make their own choices. This is why it is so important for communication with parents to be mature and transparent, providing a balanced view on the prevention of inappropriate marketing and promotion of both breastfeeding and the use of infant formula.

Integrated approach to infant and young-child diet

Breastfeeding is a single entity that must be considered within the context of other nutritive and non-nutritive factors which have an impact on the health and wellbeing of infants and children. Open and inclusive multifactorial policy-making may be more receptive to families and their healthcare professionals, which pulls together these interdependent factors. Such a holistic approach would probably be more effective at a national rather than a global level. With due diligence to global principles, individual regions and countries should assess their own level of nutritional risk and shape their infant-feeding policies to meet the broader health and social needs of families at risk. The review panels should consider whether there should be a global minimum standard for infant feeding practice that can be adjusted according to specific national risk factors. A stepwise approach like this may be more realistic for parents who are sceptical about being given the same advice whether they live in Switzerland or Sierra Leone.

Although policies and directives should be cognizant of the nutritional interdependence between breastmilk and complementary foods, research and policy tend to consider these as separate entities, whereby breastfeeding overshadows the importance of complementary foods. Paradoxically, countries with the longest duration of breastfeeding generally have the highest childhood mortality and stunting. From a nutrition perspective, this can be explained by reverse causality – the longer duration of breastfeeding reflects the lack of good-quality complementary foods in the study populations. In these circumstances breastmilk acts as an inadequate complementary food substitute. Breastmilk may be providing sufficient energy and nutrients for survival in *early* life, but the failure to simultaneously scale-up complementary feeding inevitably leads to greater mortality and morbidity among the children. It therefore needs to be appreciated that all forms of infant nutrition complement each other.

Policy integration

In the nine WHA resolutions relating to infant feeding from 2005 to 2018, breastfeeding was mentioned forty-one times; the phrase 'complementary feeding' only seven times (unpublished data). It has been postulated that breaches of the Code have fuelled policy-makers' suspicions that industry exploits opportunities to promote complementary food products and, in turn, industry has become wary of breastfeeding advocates and activists, viewing them as potentially hostile to their brand name. Consequently, they have been reluctant to play a meaningful role in scaling-up complementary products.

Instead, industry has focused on older children, with fast foods, confectionery and sugary drinks, which have contributed to the obesity component of the double burden of malnutrition. The consequences of this dysfunctional behaviour by key stakeholders are immeasurable. Although the Code was developed to limit the industry's actions and behaviours, it also limits the opportunities for other members of the infant-feeding community to work with the food industry to improve the quality of complementary feeding, and to provide a foundation for a diverse balanced diet in later childhood. The impact of the Code on health outcomes must be assessed afresh, to determine which aspects are supported by *evidence* of benefit and which areas are counterproductive and potentially damaging.

In the recent *Lancet* series on the double burden of malnutrition,[6] it was suggested that actions to address undernutrition, overweight and obesity have historically adopted a policy 'silo' approach, and there is emerging evidence that programmes addressing undernutrition have unintentionally increased the risks for obesity and diet-related non-communicable diseases in low- and middle-income countries. This provides further evidence for a more holistic approach, albeit belated, and the need for a *fully* integrated approach to *all* aspects of the infant and young-child diet.

Independent regulatory authorities

There needs to be clarity on who or what is being regulated, and by whom. Clear lines of responsibility are necessary for marketing and promotion by industry, with assessment by an independent regulatory body. Scientists and healthcare professionals are already under the jurisdiction of statutory regulatory systems, through which are channelled any concerns regarding practice or behaviour. But breastfeeding advocacy and activist groups also have to demonstrate that their organizations meet all the relevant governance standards. Families should not only be able to contribute to the development of policy proposals, but also be protected from any proposals that might be perceived as insensitive to the needs of parents and their infants. A citizens communication system, provided by an independent body, might function to provide valuable consumer data that can inform policy development. Currently the principal decision-maker is the WHA and, interestingly, it is unclear who governs the WHA.

Even with the best partnership-working, it is inevitable that claims of conflict of interest emerge. The material risk identified in a claim has to be assessed with due diligence, thus ensuring that the evaluation does not fall victim to further conflicts of interest. Blatant conflicts of interest should be easily identified, but bear in mind that any assessment of a potential conflict introduces elements of judgement and opinion rather than fact. When this happens, there may be a fine divide between good judgement, self-interest and the conflict of interest. With this degree of uncertainty, it is essential for claims of conflict of interests to be responsible and proportionate – not to be used as a tool by individuals or organizations to advance their self-interest and create yet more division and distrust.

The NetCode system initiated by WHO and breastfeeding interest groups is clearly divisive.[7] Half of the infant-feeding community is monitoring the other half, but this is not a reciprocal arrangement. It could also be argued that the *least*-regulated organizations are regulating the *most*-regulated organizations.

For a solid foundation of good practice, all organizations involved in the infant-feeding community must be able to demonstrate optimum standards relating to professionalism, governance and regulation, and they should be assessed by independent regulatory bodies. Organizations that are considered by a regulatory body not to meet such standards should not participate in policy-making.

To ensure that governance is at the heart of all decisions within the infant and young child policymaking system there needs to be an independent governance body that will provide an external oversight of the internal governance within the individual organizations. Any governance concerns should be referred to the proposed international governance board, which would have the remit to advise WHO/WHA, governments and organizations on the establishment of governance structures and systems that will underpin the Code and other relevant policies.

The way forward

The interdependent roles of breastmilk, complementary foods and formulas should, if required, be central to academic research and multi-stakeholder policy-making, with a focus on delivering an integrated, balanced nutritional diet that is specific for the age and socioeconomic circumstances of infants and young children. The only way this can be achieved is by changing the current approach, and several key determinants that have been identified in this critique could provide material evidence for a long-overdue independent review.

Leadership is the key to the successful promotion of change, and leaders need to have the confidence and support of those that are responsible for delivering change. For this to be achieved there has to be communication that allows the sharing of ideas, and the coalescence of these ideas leads to a plan that has the support of all stakeholders and engenders a sense of ownership with the target population. The immediate objective should be to change the environment of infant and young-child feeding policy from longstanding division and hostility to a future in which mutual engagement leads to collective and constructive decisions. Policy decisions should be proportionate and complementary, and the focus should be on parents and health professionals who have the day-to-day responsibility for the health and wellbeing of the child. This will require the hostile ambience around infant feeding to be desensitized and destigmatized, and for the 'milk of human kindness' to extend to all those involved in the process of policy-making and practice.

As a precedent, note that members of the WHA requested, in 2015, WHO's Director-General to establish a review committee to examine the role of international health regulations in the Ebola outbreak of 2014, and to consider WHO's response.[8] There were 28,616 cases of Ebola and 11,310 deaths across Guinea, Liberia and Sierra Leone. In 2018, there were *2.4 million* nutrition-related childhood deaths worldwide. With a background of partnership dysfunction and a failure to meet key objectives, the members of WHA should be seeking assurance on performance and governance, and this can be provided by an independent review that critically considers the strengths and limitations of the current policy-making process. This is a responsible way forward. Early life nutrition is the foundation of future health, and current evidence indicates that this jewel of human life deserves better.

Addendum

This chapter is based on a previously published article: Forsyth S (2020) Should there be a comprehensive independent review of infant feeding policy-making? *Annals of Nutrition and Metabolism* 76, 201–06. DOI: 10.1159/000508455. Available at: https://www.karger.com/Article/FullText/508455/.

References

1. Forsyth JS (2010) *International Code of Marketing of Breastmilk Substitutes* – three decades later time for hostilities to be replaced by effective national and international governance. *Archives of Diseases in Childhood* 95, 769–70.

2. Evans A (2018) *Food for thought. An independent assessment of the International Code of Marketing of Breastmilk Substitutes.* Breastfeeding Innovation Team. Available at: https://medium.com/@JustACTIONS/food-for-thought-an-independent-assessment-of-the-international-code-of-marketing-of-breast-milk-1d8d704ee612 (last accessed August 2022).

3. Grummer-Strawn LM (2019) Response to letter: confusion over breastmilk substitutes. *Journal of Pediatric Gastroenterology and Nutrition* 68(2), e41–42.

4. Forsyth S (2018) Is WHO creating unnecessary confusion over breastmilk substitutes? *Journal of Pediatric Gastroenterology and Nutrition* 67, 760–62.

5. OECD (2009) *Focus on Citizens: Public Engagement for Better Policy and Services.* ISBN 978-92-64-04886-7.

6. Branca F, Demaio A, Udomkesmalee E, *et al.* (2020) A new nutrition manifesto for a new nutrition reality. *The Lancet* 395, 8–10.

7. WHO/UN Children's Fund (2017) *NetCode toolkit. Monitoring the marketing of breastmilk substitutes: protocol for ongoing monitoring systems.* Licence CC BY-NC-SA 3.0 IGO. Available at: https://apps.who.int/iris/bitstream/handle/10665/259441/9789241513180-eng.pdf (last accessed August 2022).

8. WHO (2015) *WHO Secretariat response to the report of the Ebola Interim Assessment Panel.* Available at: https://www.who.int/csr/resources/publications/ebola/who-response-to-ebola-report.pdf (last accessed August 2022).

CHAPTER 17

A memorandum of understanding between WHO and Nestlé

To bring a resolution to so many years of conflict, to collectively address the nutritional needs of children worldwide, to encourage research and development in the area of infant and child nutrition, and to provide reassurance and support to families, there needs to be a meeting of minds and universal commitment from all key individuals and organizations. The process needs to start with a professional understanding between the two key combative players – WHO and Nestlé. If this cannot be achieved through consensus, then the only course of action will be through legal challenges in a court of law.

The consequences of longstanding mistrust and acrimony provide a significant hurdle for both parties to overcome and the option of a MoU or equivalent has been raised. This will require both parties to set aside past grievances, develop a constructive vision of their future relationship and how this will engage with the other stakeholders, and for this to evolve into a partnership that is based on trust and respect. This should allow the range of knowledge and expertise that is available in the field of infant and young child nutrition to guide a shared understanding of the best way forward. Both WHO and Nestlé must give serious consideration to what they can bring to the discussions that will unlock the current impasse in partnership-working.

What should Nestlé and WHO bring to the table?

As Nestlé is the largest food and beverage company in the world, I believe it should take the lead role within the infant and young child food industry and bring proposals that will address the key issues that have bedevilled compliance with the Code and soured relations with the other key stakeholder. I suggest that the following will be required of Nestlé to participate in the first meeting with WHO:

- A genuine commitment to resolving the longstanding issues and an acceptance that past business decisions, especially in the areas of promotion, marketing and sales of infant formulas and related products, have not served the best interests of infants, their families and other stakeholders, for which Nestlé now should apologize.
- Willingness to comply with the current Code, and subsequent versions of the Code.
- Willingness to collaborate with WHO and other stakeholders in developing policies aimed at reducing and preventing all forms of malnutrition, including the double burden of malnutrition.
- Willingness to collaborate with WHO and other stakeholders, especially academia, in pursuing research solutions to infant and child nutrition.
- Willingness to follow strict governance standards relating to collaboration with healthcare professionals in relation to guidelines on clinical practice, education and research.
- Willingness to agree to independent scrutiny of all complaints in relation to industry-related alleged breaches of the Code.
- Willingness to take a lead role in enabling all other infant-formula companies to collectively support the agreements contained within the MoU.
- Willingness to agree that their involvement in infant and young-child nutrition will be monitored by an independent regulatory authority.

And what should WHO bring to the table? These are my thoughts:

- A genuine commitment to resolving the longstanding issues and an acceptance that past decisions, especially in the areas of leadership, engagement, transparency and professional accountability, have not served the best interests of infants, their families and other stakeholders, for which WHO now should apologize.
- Willingness to ensure that the Code applies to all stakeholders, including WHO, WHA, healthcare, breastfeeding activists and industry.
- Willingness to ensure that all stakeholders, including health professionals, parents and industry collaborate in developing policies aimed at reducing and preventing all forms of malnutrition, including the double burden of malnutrition.

- Willingness to commit to regular updates of the Code with stakeholder involvement.
- Willingness to ensure that policy-making is inclusive and that recommendations will be judged by key stakeholders as realistic and achievable.
- Willingness to work closely with governments to ensure that global and national policy-making is complementary and sensitive to the needs of individual countries.
- Willingness to agree that their involvement in infant and young-child nutrition will be monitored by an independent regulatory authority

To facilitate these conditions, there needs to be a neutralization of the most significant areas of acrimony and division and there are four areas to which this might apply.

The first and the most contentious area is the alleged (and frequently confirmed) claims that industry is not complying with the Code. This usually relates to a product that they are promoting and the information on the product not complying with the regulations set out in the Code. It is usually detected once the product is on the market and available on retail shelves. It is therefore suggested that all infant-formula products and their related information need to be assessed at a global trading standards office *before* the product can go on the market. If those standards are met the product will be given a seal of approval, to be indicated on the product label. If the product does not receive a seal of approval, it would be illegal to market and sell it, and the trader would also be culpable. Any new product or modified product would be subject to this process. This validation system would set a global standard and apply to all infant-formula companies worldwide.

The second area relates to WHO's policy approach of one-size-fits-all. Parents and health professionals, in particular, find it difficult to understand why the benefits and risks of not complying with WHO breastfeeding policy are the same if you live in a high- or low-income country, despite the child mortality rate being different by at least a factor of ten. Parents want risk assessments and policies that relate to *them*, and the lack of such information is a key factor in the lack of engagement and compliance with WHO recommendations.

The third area is the need for researchers and health professionals to be able to collaborate with industry on research and educational projects – without being subjected to unsubstantiated claims of conflict of interest. It has been unfortunate that WHO officials have joined breastfeeding activist groups in adopting the view that you are guilty until proven innocent. If someone has a concern about a paediatrician, they can be referred to a regulating body (in most cases a general medical council) and will then be investigated. It is suggested that all stakeholders engaged in the policy-making process must be monitored by an independent regulatory authority. If this is not in place, they cannot participate.

Finally, there is a need to create a climate that allows constructive discussion and shared resolutions. Many things have been said and done over the last forty years to fuel the conflict, which must now be set aside, and thus clearing the way to make a meaningful step forward. An apology is a powerful way to de-escalate previous actions and challenging conversations that have featured during the conflict. It is also important to note that it is extremely rare for conflicts to start and escalate due solely to the actions of one person or group. It is therefore proposed that each stakeholder takes responsibility for their inappropriate behaviour and offers apologies to those they have failed to serve adequately. This could be included in the MoU.

Having addressed these four issues, attention can then be given to the detail of the MoU, and for illustrative purposes, a proposed MoU is outlined in Box 17.1.

Box 17.1: Infant and young-child nutrition—the importance of stakeholder participation and collaboration: A proposed memorandum of understanding (MoU)

THE VISION

The vision would encompass this statement from WHO's *International Code of Marketing of Breastmilk Substitutes* (Geneva 1981):

"Affirming the need for governments, organizations of the United Nations system, non-governmental organizations, experts in various related disciplines, consumer groups and industry to cooperate in activities aimed at the improvement of maternal, infant and young-child health and nutrition".

In 1981, the Code was viewed as a seminal policy, and few would disagree with that today. The above statement clearly indicates the importance of all stakeholders cooperating in their activities aimed at improving maternal, infant and young-child health and nutrition. At that time, it was anticipated that the Code would provide the framework for this to be achieved, however, the evidence from the last four decades indicates that the aspiration of collective

---

cooperation has not been achieved. It is therefore proposed that a potential mechanism for progressing towards more effective partnership-working within an environment of trust, respect, shared understanding, and governance, is the development of a Memorandum of Understanding.

What is a MoU?

A MoU is simply a written agreement that identifies the working relationships and guidelines between collaborating entities. It spells out common understandings, expresses a convergence of will between the parties, indicates an intended common line of action, and defines the rights and responsibilities of each entity. The essential characteristic of a MoU is that it is a *statement of intention*. It is neither legally binding nor a formal contract.

How should the MoU be structured and what should it state?

The following should be included:

- The purpose and goals of the collaboration or partnership.
- The terms of the agreement.
- The processes and procedures arising from terms of agreement.
- The procedures for modification and termination of the MoU.
- The signatories of all participating stakeholders.

What is the purpose and goal of the MoU?

The purpose and goal should be to identify areas of agreement and shared understanding that encourage and strengthen stakeholder participation and collaboration and thus allow outstanding key issues relating to infant and young-child nutrition to be effectively addressed in an environment of trust and respect.

Terms of the agreement of the MoU

POLICY-MAKING

1. A sense of mutual understanding and shared ownership across all key stakeholders.

2. A process that is conducted in a climate of trust and respect.

3. Discussions and decisions focused on the specific needs of infants, children and parents.

4. Recommendations that may be global, regional or national, depending on the potential impact of social, economic and cultural diversity.

5. Recognition of the knowledge and skills of each of the stakeholders, with the scope to contribute effectively to the policy-making process.

6. Formal engagement with consumers and practitioners as an essential part of policy development and effective implementation.

7. Policy recommendations that are sensitive, flexible and achievable, and reflect real-world settings.

8. Consideration of the totality of evidence from researchers, healthcare workers, policy-makers and other key stakeholders, relating the level of evidence to the most appropriate actions.

9. Avoidance of the context of interest groups advocating for competing recommendations based on the same evidence; the dietary needs of the most vulnerable infants must be at the centre of discussions.

10. Priority given to a continuum of high-quality diet from birth to five years, recognizing the importance of breastmilk (or infant formula), complementary feeding and young-child foods.

IMPLEMENTATION

1. Ethical principles and mutually agreed governance standards should underpin all aspects of implementation of policy.

2. Consumers and practitioners should have a key role in developing implementation plans.

3. Priority should be given to the most vulnerable populations, delivered through integrated, multi-sectoral actions facilitated by high-level political support.

4. Implementation may comprise full-scale interventions or incremental targeted developments.

5. Effective local engagement should be established to ensure there is a sense of ownership and commitment.

LEADERSHIP

1. Leadership of a multi-faceted process is complex and requires many skills including engagement integrity, and transparency.

2. WHO, WHA, UNICEF and Codex should ensure that consultation is inclusive, and that decision-making clearly reflects the views of consumers and practitioners.

3. Governments should ensure that national policy reflects the specific needs of their child population.

4. The provision of high-quality Infant and young-child nutrition must be perceived as a pleasurable and rewarding experience by all stakeholders, especially families.

RESEARCH, EDUCATION & TRAINING

1. The knowledge and skills of every stakeholder should be utilized to improve the quality of nutrition for infants and young children.

2. Collaborative research should be encouraged, and be closely monitored to ensure that ethical, scientific and governance standards are met.

3. Education about the infant and young-child diet should involve all stakeholders, especially researchers and practitioners.

4. Multidisciplinary training of all stakeholders should take place to ensure ongoing effective multi-professional working.

Processes and procedures arising from terms of agreement

The MoU should be self-regulated by the stakeholder signatories, however all stakeholders should be monitored by an independent regulatory authority.

Procedures for modification and termination of the MoU

If a stakeholder wishes to withdraw from the MoU, their decision must be accepted by the remaining signatories. The terms of agreement of any signatory may be modified with the agreement of the majority of stakeholder signatories.

Signatories of the MoU

Any stakeholder may become a signatory of the MoU. Continuing commitment to the MoU will be demonstrated by a planned renewal of the stakeholder signatory.

Process

The integration of industry into the policy-making process would need to be planned and agreed. This process would be challenging for some stakeholders, but the collaboration could be monitored by an independent committee to provide some reassurance to WHO, industry and the other stakeholders.

CHAPTER 18

A framework for change management

There are several key issues that over many years have fuelled controversy and conflict over policy-making for infant and young-child feeding, presenting an obstacle to consensus management. These issues are covered below. For each one, I have listed statements of reality and intent that might provide the steppingstones for developing a consensus management structure and function for delivering the best nutrition for infants and young children worldwide.

Global and national policy making

- Constitutionally, WHO assists governments, upon request, to strengthen health services.
- Governments have responsibility for serving the health needs of their citizens.
- The Code was adopted as a recommendation – not as a regulation.
- Significant non-compliance with implementation of the Code is evident globally.
- There is a lack of independent review of global infant-feeding policies to guide change.
- Policies need to be subject to accepted governance standards.
- Governance structures specific for each of the stakeholders need to be strengthened.

Infant feeding and morbidity and mortality

- The prevalence of breastfeeding is greatest in low-income countries.
- Low-income countries have the highest rates of infant and child mortality and morbidity.
- Low-income countries are at the greatest risk of inadequate supplies of nutritious foods.

- High-income countries have low rates of breastfeeding.
- High-income countries have significantly lower infant and young child mortality and morbidity.
- High-income countries have higher sales of infant formula.
- High-income countries have adequate supplies of nutritious foods.
- High- and low-income countries need food that is safe and nutritious.
- Infant-feeding policy must reflect the diversity of need.

Breastmilk and infant formula

- Breastfeeding is superior to infant formula.
- Infants who are not breastfed need to receive infant formula.
- Infant formulas need to reflect the best scientific and technological evidence.
- Formula development needs to be independently regulated.
- Regulation should ensure that marketing and promotion of both breastmilk and infant formulas meet agreed standards.

Complementary feeding

- The focus on breastfeeding has overshadowed the importance of complementary feeding.
- There is a suspicion that industry will exploit the opportunity to promote complementary products.
- Industry is wary of breastfeeding activists who have been hostile to their brand and business.
- Simultaneous scaling-up of breastfeeding and complementary feeding makes nutritional sense.
- The focus should be on the successful establishment of a balanced nutritional diet in early life.
- Stakeholder collaboration (including industry) on complementary feeding needs to be strengthened and monitored.

Inequality

- There are social and health inequalities between breastfed and formula-fed infants.

- Multi-agency working needs to mitigate the effects of disadvantage in formula-fed infants.
- All aspects of healthcare need to focus on reducing inequality.
- Infant formulas are a safety net for the most vulnerable infants.
- Regulation should ensure that stakeholder self-interest does not create additional inequality.

The importance of food

- Childhood obesity is most prevalent in high-income countries.
- Childhood obesity is becoming prevalent in countries classified as emerging economies.
- Infant and young-child feeding policies deter collaboration with industry.
- Food is a key determining health factor for child health in low- and high-income countries.
- *No* food, the *wrong* food and *excess* food continue to be a global health crisis in child health.
- Nutrition strategies should focus on ensuring global availability of nutritious foods.

Parental involvement

- Parents are the ultimate provider of infant feeding.
- Engagement with parents has to be balanced and sensitive to the diversity of need.
- The majority of parents are not activists, but they are pragmatists coping with the pressures of modern life.
- As the needs of a population evolve, policies must adapt to societal change.
- Compliance with infant-feeding policy requires consensus from parents.
- Consensus from parents requires consultation with parents.

Health benefits of breastfeeding for infants

- Breastfeeding is reported to provide significant health benefits for infants.
- The relationship between breastfeeding and most health conditions is 'an association'.

- With 'associations', known or unknown variables may be responsible for the link to breastfeeding.
- In these circumstances, evidence of direct cause and effect requires further investigation.
- The strengths and limitations of data and evidence must be carefully presented.
- The marketing and promotion of breastfeeding should reflect the quality of the evidence.

Infant-feeding policy

- Infant-feeding policies need to reach out to parents and their health professionals.
- Parents have to believe that the policy will serve the requirements of their children.
- The need for breastmilk, infant formula (if required), and complementary foods should be acknowledged.
- Issues relating to the timing of these dietary transitions persist.
- Both nutritive and non-nutritive factors underpin the best feeding regimen for individual infants.
- The psychosocial effects of over-reaching breastfeeding targets can create physical and emotional harm.
- A balanced incremental approach may allow a greater sense of ownership and confidence.
- Infant-feeding policy needs to deliver a successful, pleasurable and rewarding experience for parents and their children.

Conflict of interest

- Even with the best partnership-working, it is inevitable that some claims of conflict of interest will emerge.
- It is important that any claims of conflict of interest are responsible and proportionate.
- Claims of conflict of interest can be generated by underlying issues of acrimony and mistrust.
- Conflict of interest should not be used by organizations to advance self-interest.

- Good practice relies on all organizations meeting agreed governance standards.
- Conflict of interest needs to be independently regulated.

Interest groups, advocates and activists

- Interest groups have a key role to play in our society.
- Special interest and activist groups can make contributions that raise infant-feeding standards.
- Ideologists and realists should work together to determine the needs of the target population.
- All stakeholders must have a clear understanding of the value of the multidisciplinary approach.
- All stakeholders need to influence and deliver their messages within a regulated environment.
- Leadership should be inclusive and unifying.

Partnership-working

- Partnership-working is a key element of many aspects of paediatric care, including infant feeding.
- Effective partnerships strengthen governance; divided partnerships create dysfunction.
- Effective leadership needs to unify the partnership through engagement, support and respect.
- Stakeholders bring specialist knowledge and expertise to the discussion.
- The key to partnership-working is a shared understanding of the issue that is being addressed.
- The infant-feeding partnership should deliver policies that are credible, desirable and achievable.

Governance

- Multi-agency monitoring systems have failed to deliver effective corporate governance.
- All stakeholders need to be affiliated with an independent regulatory organization.

- Regulation should ensure processes meet clinical, professional and financial governance standards.
- Global decisions made by the WHA should meet agreed governance standards.
- Governments and their healthcare systems need to establish transparent governance processes.
- The delivery of optimum nutrition should be driven by governance that is proportionate and robust.
- Parental engagement should be a key governance standard for infant-feeding policies.

Critical success factors

- Effective partnership-working needs to be evidenced.
- Discussion and decision-making should be conducted in a climate of trust and respect.
- A global 'one-size-fits all' approach must be balanced with more localized and individualized nutritional care.
- Idealism and pragmatism need to converge in order to meet the needs of the silent majority.
- High-quality policy-making needs to be evidenced by professionalism, governance and regulation.

CHAPTER 19

Seven steps to transformational change

This critique has identified several areas of systemic failure that will only be resolved through significant transformational change.

Step 1: Establish a strategic framework that appropriately balances global and national responsibilities

WHO and WHA should be responsible for global leadership of infant and young-child feeding which is delivered through agreed global principles and through guidance. In addition to WHO/WHA structures there should be an independent Strategic Advisory Group (SAG) that brings together the breadth of knowledge and expertise that is required to ensure that a holistic and sensitive approach is taken to nutritional care of infants and young children worldwide. At national level, governments should embrace the global principles but be directly responsible for developing national policies, supporting practices, and monitoring progress.

Step 2: Develop a global and national code of practice for infant and young-child feeding

In relation to infant feeding practice all key stakeholders should participate in an integrated process to provide strategic recommendations on feeding standards for infants and young children. All aspects of feeding should be included, and the process should ensure that standards are coherent and routinely updated, as required. The standards will be optimally balanced between global and national responsibility, and an international governance board (IGB) should exist, with the remit to advise WHO, WHA and governments and organizations on the importance of the policy-making process adhering to established governance structures and systems that have to underpin agreed policies.

Step 3: Devise a global regulatory framework for regulation of infant formula and related products

The violations of the International Code for marketing and promotion of breastmilk substitutes should be viewed as a Trading Standards responsibility and dealt with separately from infant-feeding policy. To reduce industry violations of the Code a *specialized* global trading standards framework for all infant-feeding products should be established. This framework should:

- ensure that infant-formula products and related texts are fully assessed
- ensure the products are given a seal of approval before entering the global market
- hold approval data on a register for all relevant products globally
- agree minimum global standards
- use digital technology to allow contemporaneous information to flow across the system from initial evaluation to consumers worldwide, and in reverse to inform trading standards authorities of potential violations.

It is proposed that this is coordinated by Codex Alimentarius.

Step 4: Create a research framework that supports research in academic and industry environments

Policy and practice need to be underpinned by robust data. To prevent the repetition of flaws in design, methodology and interpretation, an independent Global Research Advisory Centre for Infant Feeding (GRACIF) should be established and would probably be affiliated to an appropriate academic centre of excellence. This centre of excellence would:

- advise researchers on the priorities for infant and young-child feeding
- share the learning from previous studies
- advise on messaging with stakeholders and other organizations
- highlight the critical elements of study design and methodology
- act as a data-monitoring and coordinating centre.

Step 5: Provide a governance framework to set standards for all stakeholders

All organizations associated with infant and young-child feeding policy-making, including WHO and WHA, need to be affiliated with an independent regulatory organization. The respective governance organizations will serve to ensure that optimum standards for professionalism, governance, and regulation are met by each of the stakeholders. Organizations that are considered by the regulatory body to not meet agreed standards, should not be allowed to participate in infant-feeding policy-making. The governance arrangements would be monitored by the International Governance Board (Step 2).

Step 6: Design a parental involvement framework

Public consultations should not be hijacked by the vociferous few within society, who may not represent the views of the silent majority. It is important to have a system through which families can communicate their views online, and this rich and more diverse source of information could then inform future policy-making. This would entail having a public communication system, served by an independent information organization, with the objective of providing more current and in-depth consumer perspectives on infant and young-child feeding.

Step 7: Draw up a memorandum of understanding (MoU) between WHO and Nestlé

For policy-making to progress in this area there needs to be resolution of the WHO and Nestlé conflict. At present this is the *"elephant in the room"* that prevents normal discussion and collaboration between key infant feeding stakeholders. It is therefore proposed that an MoU, or similar commitment, is agreed by the Director General of WHO and the Chief Executive of Nestlé. Such an agreement should be honest, insightful and apologetic, and should set out how both WHO and Nestlé (and other infant-formula companies) can constructively work together, and with other stakeholders, with the purpose of elevating infant and young-child policy-making to a position whereby the process and outcomes reflect the highest standards of scientific evidence, professionalism and organizational credibility.

CHAPTER 20

Final reflections

I graduated in medicine at Glasgow University, Scotland, in 1973, and retired from clinical practice as a consultant paediatrician in 2009. During my career I spent many hours with parents discussing the nutritional care of their infants and young children. I considered these conversations as a two-way exchange – parents hopefully learning from me, and I always learning from them. It is an accepted *modus operandi* that listening and learning are key elements for enabling change, and in relation to infant feeding, communication with parents can be insightful and discerning. It is therefore critically important not to underestimate the potential learning that can be obtained through parental instincts and good sense, especially when it comes to the management of the nutritional health and wellbeing of their infants and children.

Unfortunately, at an infant-feeding policy level, the sentiment of listening and learning from parents appears to be highly selective. This is evident from the adoption of one-size-fits-all 'top–down' global policies that are insensitive to the views of non-activist parents and their health professionals, and not surprisingly policy compliance remains low.

The commitment of WHO to the view that every mother – worldwide – will feed her infant exactly the same way as every other infant worldwide, no matter what their geographical, nutritional and socioeconomic circumstances are, is difficult for parents to comprehend. It is also perplexing for scientists and clinicians who are familiar with the scientific evidence.

It needs to be understood that the health and wellbeing of infants and young children depends on a wide range of nutritive and non-nutritive factors and it is the inter-play of these many factors that will determine eventual health outcomes. Failure to appreciate this complexity can misrepresent the evidence that relates infant and young child nutrition to early and late health outcomes.

The approach of my critique has therefore been to take a health-professional perspective, and to unpick the areas of complexity (and conflict), appraise current policies and practices, reflect on the politics, and constructively attempt to find solutions that will make infant and young-child feeding policy more credible, desirable, and achievable, and most importantly – will address parental concerns and *save children's lives*.

The complexity of the underlying issues is best illustrated by the evidence of recurring paradoxes. For example, low-income countries with the highest rates of malnutrition, wasting, stunting and child mortality (such as the sub-Saharan countries) generally have the longest durations of breastfeeding. In contrast countries with emerging economies (such as East Asia), report rapidly declining infant and child mortality rates despite increasing consumption of infant formula.

Such paradoxes can be explained by the concept of 'reverse causality', with the primary cause of adverse infant and child health being the economic status of the country, and parental decisions to breastfeed or formula feed strongly relate to the economic status of individual families.

It is interesting that in the more advanced higher-income countries infant feeding practice has tended to shift towards the middle ground, with reports of breastfeeding initiation rates increasing, and more mothers exclusively breastfeeding during the initial months, but the WHO recommendation for continuing breastfeeding for two years or beyond continues to receive minimal support.

From a policy perspective, it is therefore important to consider infant and young-child health outcomes within the context of the societal paradigm that exists within each individual country. This approach may provide guidance on the most appropriate minimum infant-feeding requirements for specific populations.

Although breastmilk is universally accepted as the optimum source of nutrition from birth, it must be appreciated that it is just one of many nutritional and non-nutritional factors that can positively influence growth and development in early life. Thus, a more rational holistic approach to infant and young-child feeding is essential. Each of the nutrition-related factors are interdependent and cumulatively they can provide greater benefit to a child and their family than any individual single component, including breastfeeding.

This is why it is so important that the WHO's enthralment with breastfeeding should not be at the expense of other valid health-rewarding interventions. And it is imperative that infant-feeding policies are critically examined to ensure that improving health and wellbeing of infants and their mothers is the *primary* objective, with each component of the policy aimed at achieving this objective.

A policy is of little value if it does not successfully engage with a target population. Because populations are heterogeneous, heterogeneity should be a key element of policy. WHO policy has tended to include statements that may accord with the views of the vociferous minority but not necessarily with that of the more moderate silent majority. Two obvious examples include the policy on breastfeeding for two years or beyond, and more recently the WHO and activist driven re-defining of the term breastmilk substitute.

Breastfeeding is the final phase of the reproductive cycle – following on from conception, placentation and parturition – so it is not surprising that breastfeeding stimulates emotions and passions that can dominate infant-feeding policy-making discussions, and lead to idealization of breastfeeding. The term 'idealization' is generally applied where overly positive qualities may be attributed to a person, object or subject. The term 'devaluation' is used to describe the opposite effect, by which overly negative qualities are applied to a person, object or subject.

With respect to infant feeding, both of these undoubtedly occur; policy-makers and activist groups have a strong tendency to idealize breastfeeding and to devalue formula feeding, whereas across other stakeholders the balance between idealization and devaluation may be more moderate.

The perception that breastfeeding is a natural biological process that can be undertaken successfully by all women is undoubtedly a major driver of the idealiz-ation of breastfeeding. However, biological systems are unfortunately not infallible, as evidenced, for example, within the reproductive system where there may be concerns and need for intervention with conception, placentation and parturition.

Interestingly, lactational difficulties are generally not presumed to be associated with biological dysfunction originating within the breast. Instead, there is a focus on external factors that may (or may not) be associated with cessation of breastfeeding. It has been known for many years in the dairy industry that genetic predisposition can modify milk production and duration of lactation, but it is only recently that scientific evidence in humans suggests that maternal genetic markers may modify mammary gland anatomy, physiology, lactation and milk composition.

A greater understanding of the effect of genetic variation and potential non-genetic modifying factors may lead to interventions that could enhance biological lactational performance and subsequently improve the health and wellbeing of infants and children. In the meantime, it is important for policy-makers and practitioners to remain sensitive to this ongoing research as a possible explanation for suboptimal lactation.

Molecular biological developments may also have relevance to the reported associations between breastfeeding and a range of health conditions. For example, they may provide an alternative narrative for the relationship between sub-optimal lactation and breast cancer.

Unless we wish to return to the late 1880s or early 1990s, when the loss of infant lives from a lack of breastmilk and the absence of a safe alternative had a devastating effect, we need to ensure that infants who are not receiving breastmilk, do have access to a safe commercial alternative, and this is acknowledged in the Code.

So it is very important for stakeholders to not only pursue policies to encourage breastfeeding, but also to be cognizant of the importance of providing the best possible safety net for infants when breastmilk is not an option. Moreover, there must be full appreciation that liquid diets have to be complemented by nutritious complementary foods which, for large sections of the global population, may not be readily available. In these circumstances, the safety net needs to be extended to the availability of commercially prepared foods that meet nutritional requirements and are packaged to ensure that consumption is safe in environments where water is unclean, sanitation is inadequate, and cooking facilities may not be accessible.

Infant and young-child feeding should therefore include a menu of food modalities which, if utilized at the right time and in the right place, can provide a safety net for infants and young children who do not receive breastmilk or home-prepared complementary foods.

As each of these modalities can play a critical nutritional role in providing nutritional care to the most disadvantaged children, research and development in this area should be prioritized rather than be devalued. Policy-makers and practitioners need to ensure that products are prescribed and utilized appropriately. Industry needs to guarantee that marketing and promotion will comply with national and global recommendations.

An overriding concern is that policy focuses on the commodities of infant feeding, rather than the individual. A predominating 'mantra' is that all stakeholders should promote, support and protect breastfeeding, whereas a more holistic and receptive response may be to ensure that all stakeholders promote, support and protect infants and young children.

Breastfeeding is one of several entities that can contribute to this goal, but health benefits will not be achieved if the other relevant factors do not effectively contribute, at the right time. For example, the immunological benefits of breastfeeding are likely to be overwhelmed by the immunosuppressive effects of severe malnutrition.

Thus, to maximize the potential health benefits of breastmilk, other factors should be simultaneously addressed, including clean water, sanitation, housing, foods, education, health and income. For this reason, infant feeding is not *all about breastfeeding*.

The WHO is the global lead for health. It needs to provide leadership that encourages collaboration and prevents damaging divisions within the critically important area of child public health. Regrettably, in addition to the longstanding conflict with industry, WHO has in more recent times extended critical comments to paediatricians in the columns of the journals *The Lancet* and the *British Medical Journal* with regard to their professional relationship with industry. WHO has imposed on parents an unrealistic 'clarification' on what is a breastmilk substitute, and what is a complementary food. WHO has also surprisingly attempted to undermine credible opinions published by the European Food Safety Authority (EFSA) on issues relating to the nutritional composition of infant formulas, the timing of the introduction of complementary foods, and governance standards for members participating on EFSA panels. More recently, WHO representatives have clashed with Codex Alimentarius on the use of the term breastmilk substitutes.

Underlying these disputes is WHO's overwhelming commitment to breastfeeding and their desire for all countries to agree on more strict legislation to control the marketing of breastmilk substitutes. However, this will not be possible if a legally binding definition of the term 'breastmilk substitutes' cannot be agreed, and this is now in a state of flux following WHO's attempt to depart from the definition set out in the Code.

Conflict of interest is a tool that is increasingly being used by WHO and breastfeeding activist groups to fuel the 'blame culture' across the infant-feeding community. However, there is a need for WHO to reflect on their own practice in relation to conflict of opinion. WHO officials frequently conclude their published contributions by declaring:

> *"The authors alone are responsible for the views expressed in this letter and they do not necessarily represent the views, decisions, or policies of WHO. We declare no competing interests".*

This is surprising as they are employed and remunerated by WHO. They have been producing papers and working documents in relation to the Code and subsequent resolutions that have been endorsed by WHA. So, it would therefore be very odd if their views did *not* represent the views of WHO. However, if that *is* the case then there is a need for clarity on which views do – or do not – represent the views of WHO – which views are official WHO business and which views are personal to the freelancing officials? Only then can responsibility and accountability for the statements be formally attributed.

It is also important to note that material conflict of interest does not have to be financial in origin to be considered unprofessional or highly damaging. Probably the most damaging conflict of interest within infant-feeding policy-making is a deep-seated prejudice against one or more stakeholders, which divides partnership-working and places unacceptable risk on the vulnerable populations they are contracted to serve.

Policies that fuel a hostile and persistent blame culture are failed policies. And policy-makers need to reconstruct these policies in order to align achievable objectives with avoidance of blame. This necessitates that all key stakeholders should contribute to, and take responsibility for, the endorsed policy. However, with their current orientation, it is difficult to see how WHO can deliver an effective multi-stakeholder approach to nutritional policymaking, *without* committing to significant philosophical and organizational change.

If it is possible to distil this longstanding public-health conflict down to one specific point that ignited and has maintained the flames for many decades, the most obvious candidate is the failure to successfully resolve the issue of recurring violations of the Code. The purpose of the Code was to prevent inappropriate marketing and promotion of infant formulas by industry – a *bona fide* consideration that is generally supported. However, the Code also focuses on recommendations for health services, health professionals and non-activist parents, and these statements tend to relate more to the marketing and promotion of breastfeeding.

Then there is the role of WHO, WHA and breastfeeding activist groups who were the driving force for the development of the Code and responsible for much of the content, which presumably explains why there are no specific articles in the Code relating to their role and function. It is also not surprising that they are collectively the most resistant to any review of the Code.

It is therefore evident that, beyond the issues relating directly to industry, the Code is a highly contested document. Rather than focus on the single issue of industry violations, there is an unhelpful ambiguity with attention being diverted to infant-feeding practice. This leads to uncertainty as to whether this is a Code of marketing of breastmilk substitutes or whether it is a Code of marketing of breastfeeding. With the Code recommending legislation and sanctions to prevent violations it is important that this is focused on industry induced violations, and that the interests of health professionals and parents are considered separately within the infant feeding community.

To unpick the current toxic situation the following viewpoints should be considered:

- The Code document extends beyond the fundamental issue – that the inappropriate marketing and promotion of infant formulas is primarily an industry issue and the solution should lie with industry.

- The violation by industry is a breach of trading standards, which needs to be investigated and managed by trading standards and other appropriate authorities.

- The Code unnecessarily diverts attention away from industry and makes recommendations on the practice of other stakeholders, especially health professionals, health services and parents, and these recommendations should be addressed through infant-feeding policymaking where proposals relating to accepted practice can be considered and evidenced in line with all other aspects of infant-feeding policy.

- The detail of a new approach to industry violations should be set out in a new *International Code of Marketing of Breastmilk Substitutes*, and the document should focus exclusively on the operational and regulatory systems that will prevent industry from violating the marketing and promotion of their products.

- Separating industry-related violations from concerns regarding clinical practice will allow a sharper focus on the specific issue of industry violation, and ensure that clinical practice does not become a victim of recommendations that should be more specific to the inappropriate behaviour of industry.

- To provide appropriate leadership it is suggested that Codex Alimentarius, which is part of the UN family and has responsibility for protecting consumer health and ensuring fair practices in the food trade, should have overall responsibility for monitoring compliance with the infant-formula trading standards.

- WHO and national governments should continue to oversee infant-feeding policy and ensure that the needs of infants who are not breastfed, and those who need a specialised formula for a specific medical need, receive the best possible nutritional care.

The failure of WHO/WHA to review the Code over a period of more than forty years, especially when it has been the source of continuing debate and discontent, should be viewed as a major breach of institutional governance.

As the positions of the key groups become more entrenched, there does not appear to be a governance system that can take control and advise on the necessity for organizational change.

Infant-feeding discussions, especially on matters relating to breastfeeding, should not adopt positions of ideological certainty and close the door on questions of doubt.

Policymakers and interest groups need to be sensitive to the uncertainty that is common in *all* aspects of healthcare and be more receptive to expressions of doubt that could be the catalyst for a more collective understanding of the key issues.

With this imperative, this critique has identified several transformational changes that could provide the foundations for effective delivery of policy on infant and young-child feeding, and which would ultimately save children's lives. The key areas for change relate to:

- clarity on global and national responsibilities
- the requirement for codes of practice to be contemporaneous
- the need for high-quality research undertaken in academic and industry environments
- the strengthening of global regulatory systems for marketing and promotion of milk products
- the establishment of independent governance arrangements for all stakeholders, and
- the development of a framework for parental involvement.

With the increasing dysfunctionality within the infant-feeding community, and with the conflict between WHO and the infant-formula industry being the dominant issue, urgent action is required.

A bold and meaningful *first* step would be to reach an agreement on professional working relationships between WHO and industry with the Director-General of WHO and the Chief Executive of Nestlé taking the lead. It is suggested that this could be developed through a commitment to a Memorandum of Understanding.

During the Covid-19 pandemic, the Director-General of WHO strongly encouraged collaboration between scientists, clinicians and industry, emphasizing the underlying need to share their knowledge and skills to develop vaccines and medicines to eradicate the infection and save lives. The subsequent development of highly effective vaccines has been heralded as a triumph for both academia and industry. This success demonstrates how powerful collaboration can be – if key actors are allowed to undertake their work without hindrance from acrimony, division and prejudice, and (of course) if there is also adequate funding.

In contrast, infant feeding has been dominated by unacceptable dysfunctional behaviour by key stakeholders – and so much human suffering could have been prevented. A generation of wasted children and wasted lives should weigh heavily upon those who have been party to the wasted years of dysfunctional behaviour.

The impact that this longstanding, polarized and conflicted atmosphere may have had at the level of communities and families – and how this may have undermined the objective of providing the best care for individual children – should not be underestimated.

Moreover, over the last forty years, during which WHO has adopted a policy of non-cooperation with the infant and young-child food industry and has taken measures to prevent stakeholder collaboration with industry, we have witnessed the emergence of a global pandemic of childhood obesity.

In relation to the development and consequences of this public health catastrophe, the breakdown in professional relationships between global policy-makers and global infant and young-child food producers must be examined.

As stated in the introduction to this book, the thesis for my critique was that poor leadership and ineffective partnership-working are responsible for the failure to deliver infant and young-child feeding policies and practices that reflect the best scientific evidence, that meet the clinical needs of infants and young children worldwide, that are sensitive to the requirements of families living in the most diverse circumstances, and are the product of due diligence conducted within a robust governance and regulatory structure.

I have provided evidence in support of my thesis, and this reinforces the need for a formal independent review that focuses on policy, practice, leadership and governance. There is no doubt that a rigorous independent inquiry will wish to relate global outcomes in infant and child health to the performance of the key stakeholders who were given responsibility to protect and support the nutritional care of these vulnerable children.

The likelihood is that no stakeholders will escape criticism, and that blame will fall heavily upon WHO, industry and breastfeeding activist groups, whose inflexible behaviour and self-interest will be key elements of the investigation.

This critique identified many systemic deficiencies and has provided proposals for improvement, but the longstanding behaviours of individuals and organizations have left an indelible mark on this vital area of global public health. To prevent further unnecessary suffering, the wasted years must end. A fresh start must begin. And this will require new thinking, new priorities and new people.

CHAPTER 21

On the 40th anniversary of the adoption of the Code

On the 20 May 2021, a joint statement was issued by UNICEF's Executive Director Henrietta Fore and WHO's Director-General Dr Tedros Adhanom Ghebreyesus. This was at the 40th anniversary of the adoption of the Code.[1] Their initial statement read:

"In 1981, health officials from around the world gathered at the World Health Assembly to address aggressive marketing tactics by the infant and young-child feeding industry, which was promoting formula feeding over breastfeeding and causing a dramatic increase in infant morbidity and mortality. The result was the International Code of Marketing of Breastmilk Substitutes (the Code), a landmark policy framework designed to stop commercial interests from damaging breastfeeding rates and endangering the health and nutrition of the world's youngest inhabitants".

They subsequently stated that:

"On the 40th anniversary of the Code, UNICEF and WHO call on governments, health workers, and the baby food industry to fully implement and abide by the Code requirements:

- *Governments must enact and enforce legislation to prevent commercial interests from undermining breastfeeding, optimal infant and young-child feeding, and the health of children and women, including during pregnancy and breastfeeding.*

- *Health workers must protect, promote and support breastfeeding; they must not accept sponsorship from companies that market foods for infants and young children for scholarships, awards, grants, meetings, or events.*

- *The infant and young-child feeding industry must publicly commit to full compliance, globally, with the International Code of Marketing of Breastmilk Substitutes and subsequent relevant World Health Assembly resolutions".*

With this statement reiterating the content of the 1981 Code, it is evident that WHO and UNICEF do not see the need for the 40th Anniversary of the Code to provide an opportunity to revisit the original concept, to reflect on progress, to invite new thinking and to consider how a revised Code could impact more effectively on 21st-century nations worldwide, especially when the declared achievements are far from convincing. For example, the statement referred to two achievements of the Code, the first of which was:

> *"In the last four decades, there has been a 50 per cent increase in the prevalence of exclusive breastfeeding. As a result, an estimated 900 million infants globally have enjoyed the survival, growth and development benefits of exclusive breastfeeding in infancy".*

According to the current WHO data at the time of the statement, only 41% of infants are exclusively breastfed for six months. Applying this figure to the stated 50% increase in exclusive breastfeeding over the last forty years, the math suggests that the prevalence of exclusive breastfeeding probably increased from 27% to 41% during the forty years. This is the equivalent a 0.35% increase per year, and at this rate achievement of 100% exclusive breastfeeding will take more than a further hundred years. Moreover, between 1981 and 2021 there was an average of 140 million births per year. Therefore, collectively, 5600 million infants were born during the forty-year period, which indicates that the aforementioned 900 million infants account for just 16% of the infants who may have received the benefits of exclusive breastfeeding during this time.

In relation to implementation of the Code it is stated that:

> *"The majority of countries have enacted legislation to implement at least some provisions of the Code, but only 25 countries have implemented measures that are substantially aligned with the Code".*

Information on implementation of the Code shows that after forty years no country is yet fully aligned with the Code and substantial alignment has been achieved in only 12.7% of the one hundred and ninety-seven countries worldwide.2

Although the intention of WHO and UNICEF was to celebrate progress over the previous forty years, the evidence in their statements is clearly not encouraging, and their reluctance to independently review the Code will only prolong the current uncertainties and suspicions. For example:

- The practice of 'clarifying' aspects of the Code through random 'subsequent resolutions' lacks credibility because they do not command the same attention and consultation that a revised Code would attract. Moreover, observers who are more sceptical may perceive this as a tactic by WHO officials to change meaning of the Code without going down the path of a formal consultation.[3]

- The credibility of this bureaucratic balancing act may be acceptable for minor adaptations relating to the Code, but when applied to something as fundamental as the *definition of a breastmilk substitute* – a term included in the title of the Code – it is not surprising that questions continue to be asked on matters of transparency, due diligence and integrity.[4]

- Trust and respect are crucial commodities in partnership-working, and they can only be achieved if *all* partners listen and learn, and collectively reach the best solutions for the nutrition of all infants worldwide.

- It is noted that the webinar associated with the statement was sponsored by the Global Breastfeeding Collective, which includes UNICEF, WHO and twenty-five international breastfeeding support agencies. I find it perplexing that the other key aspects of infant diet are persistently overshadowed by breastfeeding, *especially* complementary feeding, which is critical for normal growth and development, and getting it wrong leads to deficiencies that result in wasting, stunting and death.

- The health benefits of breastfeeding are undermined if infants are affected negatively by other nutritive and non-nutritive deficiencies. Thus, the best outcomes will be forthcoming only when these key interdependencies are addressed simultaneously.

- A holistic infant-feeding collective that acknowledges the inter-dependency of all nutritive and non-nutritive factors in infant feeding may not only enhance health and wellbeing worldwide, but also depolarize the acrimony and division that has dominated infant-feeding policy and practice for a regretfully very long time.[5]

- Denying a new generation of parents, health professionals, scientists, policy-makers and (of course) experts from the food industry with expertise in food science, food security and food distribution, to have an opportunity to voice their opinion on the forty-year-old Code is a defiant and dangerous attitude that places at risk the nutritional health and wellbeing of infants and young children in the twenty-first century.

References

1. WHO/UNICEF (2021) Statement on the 40th anniversary of the *International Code of Marketing of Breastmilk Substitutes*. Available at: https://www.who.int/news/item/21-05-2021-WHO-UNICEF-statement-on-the-40th-anniversary-of-the-international-code-of-marketing-breastmilk-substitutes (last accessed August 2022).

2. Forsyth S (2021) 40th anniversary of the *International Code of Marketing of Breastmilk Substitutes*. *The Lancet* 398, 1042.

3. UNICEF (2021) *Infant and young-child feeding*. Available at: https://data.unicef.org/topic/nutrition/infant–and–young–child–feeding/ (last accessed August 2022).

4. UN Population Division (2019 Revision) *Future population growth*. Available at: https://ourworldindata.org/grapher/births–and–deaths–projected–to–2100?country=~OWID_WRL (last accessed August 2022).

5. Forsyth JS (2010) *International Code of Marketing of Breastmilk Substitutes* – three decades later time for hostilities to be replaced by effective national and international governance. *Archives of Diseases in Childhood* 95, 769–70.

Epilogue

The writing of this critique was concluded following the inauguration of the new President of the United States, where the call for unity was the centre-piece of all contributions, none more so than through the words of Amanda Gorman, the 22-year-old National Youth Poet Laureate. She radiated joy, conviction and purpose as she declaimed the words of her poem *The Hill We Climb*. I respectfully borrow some of her words to end this critique.

> *"And so we lift our gazes not to what stands between us, but what stands before us. We close the divide because we know, to put our future first, we must first put our differences aside. We lay down our arms so we can reach out our arms to one another. We seek harm to none and harmony to all."*

References

Agency for Healthcare, Research and Quality Effective Healthcare Program (2010) *Methods guide for effectiveness and comparative effectiveness reviews: Selecting observational studies for comparing medical interventions.* Available at: https://www.effectivehealthcare.ahrq.gov/search-for-guides-reviews-and-reports/?pageaction=displayProduct&productID=454 1509/ (last accessed August 2022).

Azad MB, Nickel NC, Bode L, *et al.* (2021) Breastfeeding and the origins of health: Interdisciplinary perspectives and priorities. *Maternal and Child Nutrition* 17, e13109.

Baby Milk Action (2012) *IBFAN's concerns regarding FTSE4Good Breastmilk Substitutes criteria, assessment process and the BMS Committee (updated 8 March 2012).* Available at: http://info.babymilkaction.org/sites/info.babymilkaction.org/files/IBFANtoFTSE%20080312.pdf (accessed September 2022).

Baby Milk Action (2016) *Resolution WHA 69.9 tackling inappropriate marketing adopted.* See: http://www.babymilkaction.org/archives/9771 (last accessed August 2022).

Baby Milk Action (2019) *EFSA's faulty consultation on the age of introduction of baby foods closes.* Available at: http://www.babymilkaction.org/archives/21087 (last accessed August 2022).

Ballardini N, Kramer MS, Oken E, *et al.* (2019) Associations of atopic dermatitis and asthma with child behaviour: results from the PROBIT cohort. *Clinical and Experimental Allergy* 49, 1235–44. DOI: 10.1111/cea.13417.

Bognar Z, De Luca D, Domellöf M, *et al.* (2020) Promoting breastfeeding and interaction of pediatric associations with providers of nutritional products. *Frontiers in Pediatrics* 8, 562870. DOI: 10.3389/fped.2020.562870.

Boss M, Gardner H, Hartmann P (2018) Normal human lactation: closing the gap. *F1000 Research 7F1000 Faculty Review* 8019.

Branca F, Demaio A, Udomkesmalee E, *et al.* (2020) A new nutrition manifesto for a new nutrition reality. *The Lancet* 395, 8–10.

Burr GO, Burr MM (1929) A new deficiency disease produced by the rigid exclusion of fat from the diet. *Journal of Biological Chemistry* 82, 345–67.

Castenmiller J, de Henauw S, Hirsch-Ernst K, *et al.* (European Food Safety Authority NDA Panel) (2019) Scientific Opinion on the appropriate age range for introduction of complementary feeding into an infant's diet. *EFSA Journal* 17, 5780.

Chew M, Brizzell C, Abbasi K, Godlee F (2014) Medical journals and industry ties. *British Medical Journal* 349, g7197.

Codex Alimentarius (2017) *Guidelines on formulated complementary foods for older infants and young children. CAC/GL 8–1991. Adopted in 1991. Amended in 2017. Revised in 2013.* Available at: https://www.fao.org/fao–who–codexalimentarius/sh–proxy/zh/?lnk=1&url=https%253A%252F%252Fworkspace.fao.org%252Fsites%252Fcodex%252FStandards%252FCXG%2B8–1991%252FCXG_008e.pdf (last accessed August 2022).

Codex Alimentarius International Food Standards. Website homepage. Available at: https://www.fao.org/fao-who-codexalimentarius/publications/en/ (last accessed August 2022).

Costello A, Branca F, Rollins N, *et al.* (2017) Health professional associations and industry funding. *The Lancet* 389, 597–98.

Cuthbertson WFJ (1999) Evolution of infant nutrition. *British Journal of Nutrition* 81, 359–71.

Dattilo AM, Carvalho RS, Feferbaum R, Forsyth S, Zhao A (2020) Hidden realities of infant feeding: systematic review of qualitative findings from parents. *Behavioural Sciences (Basel)* 10, 83.

Der G, Batty D, Deary IJ (2006) Effect of breastfeeding on intelligence in children. prospective study, sibling pairs analysis, and meta-analysis. *British Medical Journal* 4, 333(7575), 945. Available at: https://www.ncbi.nlm.nih.gov/pmc/articles/PMC1633819/pdf/bmj33300945.pdf (last accessed August 2022).

Dror K, Allen LH (2018) Overview of nutrients in human milk. *Advances in Nutrition* 9, 278S–94S.

Dugdale AE (1986) Evolution and infant feeding. *The Lancet* 1, 670–73.

EFSA (2018) *EFSA rules on competing interest management.* Available at: https://www.efsa.europa.eu/sites/default/files/corporate_publications/files/competing_interest_management_17.pdf (last accessed August 2022).

EFSA Scientific opinion (2009) DHA and ARA and visual development. Scientific substantiation of a health claim related to docosahexaenoic acid (DHA) and arachidonic acid (ARA) and visual development pursuant to Article 14 of EC Regulation No 1924/20061. Scientific Opinion of the Panel on Dietetic Products, Nutrition and Allergies (Question No EFSA-Q-2008–211). Adopted on 22 January 2009. *EFSA Journal* 941, 1–4.

Evans A (2018) *Food for thought. An independent assessment of the International Code of Marketing of Breastmilk Substitutes.* Breastfeeding Innovation Team. Available at: https://medium.com/@JustACTIONS/food-for-thought-an-independent-assessment-of-the-international-code-of-marketing-of-breast-milk-1d8d704ee612 (last accessed April 2022).

Fabian CJ, Kimler BF, Hursting SD (2015) Omega-3 fatty acids for breast cancer prevention and survivorship. *Breast Cancer Research* 17, 62. Available at: https://medium.com/@JustACTIONS/food-for-thought-an-independent-assessment-of-the-international-code-of-marketing-of-breast-milk-1d8d704ee612 (last accessed August 2022).

Fallon VM, Harrold JA, Chisholm A (2019) The impact of the UK Baby Friendly Initiative on maternal and infant health outcomes: A mixed-methods systematic review. *Maternal and Child Nutrition* 153, e12778.

FEED (2020) *The provision of infant formula at food banks in the UK*. Available at: https://static1.squarespace.com/static/5efa4a95af311446a53c8cab/t/5fd0990c5347e801a823f769/1607506207266/Feed+report+on+formula+at+foodbanks+-+December+9th+2020.pdf (last accessed August 2022).

Fewtrell M, Bronsky I, Campoy C, *et al.* (2017) Complementary feeding: A position paper by the ESPGHAN Committee on Nutrition. *Journal of Paediatric Gastroenterology and Nutrition* 64, 119–32.

Fewtrell M, Wilson DC, Booth I, *et al.* (2010) Six months of exclusive breastfeeding: how good is the evidence? *British Medical Journal* 342, c5955. DOI: 10.1136/bmj.c5955.

Flohr C, Henderson AJ, Kramer MS, *et al.* (2018) Effect of an intervention to promote breastfeeding on asthma, lung function, and atopic eczema at age 16 years: follow-up of the PROBIT randomized trial. *Journal of the American Medical Association Pediatrics* (1721), e174064. DOI: 10.1001/jamapediatrics.2017.4064. Available at: https://pubmed.ncbi.nlm.nih.gov/29131887/ (last accessed August 2022).

Forsyth JS (2010) *International Code of Marketing of Breastmilk Substitutes* – three decades later time for hostilities to be replaced by effective national and international governance. *Archives of Diseases in Childhood* 95, 769–70.

Forsyth JS (2011) Policy and pragmatism in breastfeeding. *Archives of Diseases in Childhood* 96, 909–10.

Forsyth JS, Ogston SA, Clark A, *et al.* (1993) Relation between early introduction of solid food to infants and their weight and illnesses during the first two years of life. *British Medical Journal* 306, 1572–76.

Forsyth S (2012) FTSE, WHO Code and the infant-formula industry. *Annals of Nutrition and Metabolism* 60, 154–56. DOI: 10.1159/000337304.

Forsyth S (2012) Why are we undertaking DHA supplementation studies in infants who are not DHA-deficient? *British Journal of Nutrition* 108, 948.

Forsyth S (2013) Non-compliance with the *International Code of Marketing of Breastmilk Substitutes* is not confined to the infant-formula industry. *Journal of Public Health* 35, 185–90.

Forsyth S (2015) The *British Medical Journal* should not take the law into its own hands on competing interests. *British Medical Journal* 350, g7766. Available at: https://www.bmj.com/content/350/bmj.g7766 (last accessed August 2022).

Forsyth S (2018) Dietary docosahexaenoic acid and arachidonic acid in early life: what is the best evidence for policymakers? *Annals of Nutrition and Metabolism* 72, 210–22.

Forsyth S (2018) Is WHO creating unnecessary confusion over breastmilk substitutes? *Journal of Pediatric Gastroenterology and Nutrition* 67, 760–62.

Forsyth S (2018) Should the World Health Organization relax its policy of non-cooperation with the infant food industry? *Annals of Nutrition and Metabolism* 73, 160–62.

Forsyth S (2019) Is WHO creating unnecessary confusion over breastmilk substitutes? *Journal of Pediatric Gastroenterology and Nutrition*, 68, e41.

Forsyth S (2019) Formula milk studies couldn't exist without industry. *British Medical Journal* 364, l367.

Forsyth S (2019) Infant feeding and conflict of interest: a healthcare perspective. *Annals of Nutrition and Metabolism* 75, 252–55. DOI: 10.1159/000504775.

Forsyth S (2019) What is opinion and what is evidence? *British Medical Journal* 366, l5395.

Forsyth S (2020) Should there be a comprehensive independent review of infant feeding policy-making? *Annals of Nutrition and Metabolism* 76, 201-206. DOI: 10.1159/000508455. Available at: https://www.karger.com/Article/FullText/508455/ (last accessed August 2022).

Forsyth S (2021) 40th anniversary of the *International Code of Marketing of Breastmilk Substitutes*. *The Lancet* 398, 1042.

Forsyth S (2021) Marketing of breastmilk substitutes revisited: new ideas for an old problem. *World Review of Nutrition and Dietetics* 124, 1–6. DOI: 10.1159/000516724.

Forsyth S (2022) Marketing of breast-milk substitutes revisited: new ideas for an old problem. *World Review of Nutrition and Dietetics* 124, 151–56. DOI: 10.1159/000516724.

Forsyth S, Gautier S, Salem N Jr (2017) Dietary intakes of arachidonic acid and docosahexaenoic acid in early life – with a special focus on complementary feeding in developing countries. *Annals of Nutrition and Metabolism* 70, 217–27.

FTSE Index Company (2011) *FTSE Group leads collaboration to improve breastmilk substitute marketing practices media information*. Available at: https://www.ftserussell.com/press/ftse-group-leads-collaboration-improve-breast-milk-substitute-marketing-practices (last accessed August 2022).

FTSE4Good (2011) *A note on the new FTSE4Good breastmilk substitute (BMS) marketing criteria and its impact on the FTSE4Good March 2011 Review.* Available at: https://research.ftserussell.com/products/downloads/FTSE4Good_Web_Update_March_2011.pdf (last accessed August 2022).

FTSE4Good (2017) *Inclusion criteria for the marketing of breastmilk substitutes.* Available at: https://research.ftserussell.com/products/downloads/F4G_BMS_Criteria.pdf (last accessed April 2022).

Galipeau R, Baillot A, Trottier A, Lemire L (2018) Effectiveness of interventions on breastfeeding self-efficacy and perceived insufficient milk supply: A systematic review and meta-analysis. *Maternal and Child Nutrition* 14, e12607.

Godlee F (2014) Medical journals and industry ties. *British Medical Journal* 349, g7197.

Godlee F (2018) Disentangling ourselves from 'Big Formula'. *British Medical Journal* 363, k5146.

Golan Y, Assaraf YG (2020) Genetic and physiological factors affecting human milk production and composition. *Nutrients* 12, 1500.

Greiner T (2000) *The history and importance of the Innocenti Declaration.* Available at: http://arnone.de.unifi.it/mami/congresso/greiner.pdf (last accessed August 2022).

Grummer-Strawn LM (2019) Response to letter: confusion over breastmilk substitutes. *Journal of Pediatric Gastroenterology and Nutrition* 68(2), e41–42.

Grummer-Strawn LM (2018) Clarifying the definition of breastmilk substitutes. *Journal of Pediatric Gastroenterology and Nutrition* 67, 683.

Grummer-Strawn LM (2018) Invited commentary. *Journal of Pediatric Gastroenterology and Nutrition* r6, 683. DOI: 10.1097/MPG.0000000000002137).

Grummer-Strawn LM, Holliday F, Jungo KT, Rollins N (2019) Sponsorship of national and regional professional paediatrics associations by companies that make breastmilk substitutes: evidence from a review of official websites. *BMJ Open* 9, e029035.

Harbron J, Booley S, Najaar B, Day CE (2013) Responsive feeding: establishing healthy eating behaviour early on in life. *South African Journal of Clinical Nutrition* 26 (*Suppl*) S141–49.

Harder T, Bergmann R, Kallischnigg G, Plagemann A (2005) Duration of breastfeeding and risk of overweight: a meta-analysis. *American Journal of Epidemiology* 162, 397–403. DOI:10.1093/aje/kwi222.

Hardy BJ of the Ethical, Social, and Cultural Program for Global Health, Sandra Rotman Centre, Toronto, Canada. Getting to compliance. Multisector dialogue, collaboration and the international code of marketing of breastmilk substitutes. *Journal of Public Health (Oxf)* 2013, (352) 191–92. DOI: 10.1093/pubmed/fdt025/. Available at: https://pubmed.ncbi.nlm.nih.gov/23543796/ (last accessed August 2022).

Hoddinott P, Craig LCA, Britten J, *et al.* (2012) A serial qualitative interview study of infant feeding experiences. *BMJ Open* 2, e000504. Available at: DOI:10.1136/https://bmjopen.bmj.com/content/bmjopen/2/2/e000504.full.pdf/ (last accessed August 2022).

Horta BL, Victora CG (2013) *Long-term effects of breastfeeding. A systematic review. World Health Organization.* Available at: http://apps.who.int/iris/bitstream/handle/10665/79198/9789241505307_eng.pdf;jsessionid=FFD92C1D1EFD8158876D7E831A761C55?sequence=1(last accessed August 2022).

Howie PW, Forsyth S, Ogston SA, *et al.* (1990) Protective effect of breastfeeding against infection. *British Medical Journal* 300, 11–16.

IBFAN (2014) *The advantages, disadvantages and risks of ready-to-use foods. Breast-feeding Briefs No. 56/57.* Available at: http://ibfan.org/breastfeedingbreafs/BB%2056-57-The%20advantages-disadvantages-and-risks-of-ready-to-use%20foods.pdf (last accessed February 2022).

ILSI Europe. Website homepage available at: https://ilsi.eu/(last accessed August 2022).

Innocenti declaration on the protection, promotion and support of breastfeeding (1990). Available at: https://worldbreastfeedingweek.org/2018/wp-content/uploads/2018/07/1990-Innocenti-Declaration.pdf (last accessed August 2022).

Innocenti declaration on infant and young-child feeding (2005). Available at: http://www.unicef.org/programme/breastfeeding/innocenti.htm (last accessed August 2022).

Ip S, Chung M, Raman G, *et al.* (2007) Breastfeeding and maternal and infant health outcomes in developed countries. Evidence Report/Technology Assessment No. 153. AHRQ Publication No. 07-E007 April 2007. *Evidence Report Technology Assessment* 153, 1–186.

Jackson L, De Pascalis L, Harrold J, Fallon V (2021) Guilt, shame, and postpartum infant feeding outcomes: A systematic review. *Maternal and Child Nutrition* 17, e13141.

Jasani B, Simmer K, Patole SK, Rao SC (2017) Long-chain polyunsaturated fatty acid supplementation in infants born at term (Review). *Cochrane Database of Systematic Reviews* 3, CD000376. DOI: 10.1002/14651858.CD000376.pub4.

Kelleher SL, Gagnon A, Riveraet OC, *et al.* (2019) Milk-derived miRNA profiles elucidate molecular pathways that underlie breast dysfunction in women with common genetic variants in *SLC30A2. Sci Reports* 9, 12686 Available at: https://www.ncbi.nlm.nih.gov/pmc/articles/PMC6722070 (last accessed August 2022).

Kesselheim AS, Robertson CT, Myers JA, *et al.* (2012) A randomized study of how physicians interpret research funding disclosures. *New England Journal of Medicine* 367, 1119–27.

Koletzko S, Niggemann B, Arato A, *et al.* (2012) Diagnostic approach and management of cow's milk. ESPGHAN GI Committee Practical Guidelines. *Journal of*

Pediatric Gastroenterology and Nutrition: August 55(2), 221–29. Available at: https://journals.lww.com/jpgn/Fulltext/2012/08000/Diagnostic_Approach_and_ Management_of_Cow_s_Milk.28.aspx/ (last accessed August 2022).

Kramer MS, Chalmers B, Hodnett ED, *et al.* (2001) Promotion of breastfeeding intervention trial (PROBIT): a randomized trial in the Republic of Belarus. *Journal of the American Medical Association* 285, 413–20. Available at: https://pubmed.ncbi. nlm.nih.gov/11242425/ (last accessed August 2022).

Kramer MS, Kakuma R (2002) Optimal duration of exclusive breastfeeding. *Cochrane Database of Systematic Reviews* 20128, CD003517. DOI: 10.1002/14651858.CD003517. PMID: 11869667. Available at: https://pubmed.ncbi.nlm.nih.gov/11869667/ (last accessed August 2022).

Kramer MS, Kakuma R (2012) Optimal duration of exclusive breastfeeding. *Cochrane Database of Systematic Reviews* CD003517. DOI: 10.1002/14651858.CD003517.pub2. PMID: 22895934.

Kramer MS, Matush L, Vanilovich I, *et al.* (2009) A randomized breastfeeding promotion intervention did not reduce child obesity in Belarus. *Journal of Nutrition* 139, 417S–21S. DOI: 10.3945/jn.108.097675. Available at: https://pubmed.ncbi.nlm.nih.gov/ 19106322/?from_term=Martin+RM+bELARUS&from_pos=10 (last accessed August 2022).

Lee K (2009) Understandings of global health governance: The contested landscape. In: Kay A, Williams OD (eds) *Global Health Governance: Crisis, Institutions and Political Economy.* Palgrave Macmillan. DOI: 10.1057/9780230249486_2.

Lee S, Kelleher SL (2016) Biological underpinnings of breastfeeding challenges: the role of genetics, diet, and environment on lactation physiology. *American Journal of Physiology Endocrinology and Metabolism* 311, E405–22. DOI:10.1152/ ajpendo.00495.2015.

Leong C, Howlett M (2017) On credit and blame: disentangling the motivations of public policy decision-making behaviour. *Policy Science* 50, 599–618. Available at: https://link.springer.com/content/pdf/10.1007/s11077-017-9290-4.pdf (last accessed August 2022).

Louis-Jacques A, Stuebe A (2018) Long-term maternal benefits of breastfeeding. *Contemporary Obstetrics and Gynecolology* 64(7), 26–29. Available at: https://www. contemporaryobgyn.net/view/long-term-maternal-benefits-breastfeeding (last accessed August 2022).

Lucas A, Morley R (1994) Does early nutrition in infants born before term programme later blood pressure? *British Medical Journal* 309, 304–08.

Lucas A, Morley R, Cole TJ, *et al.* (1992) Breast milk and subsequent intelligence quotient in children born preterm. *The Lancet* 339, 261–64.

Martin RM, Kramer MS, Patel R, *et al.* (2017) Effects of promoting long-term, exclusive breastfeeding on adolescent adiposity, blood pressure, and growth trajectories: a secondary analysis of a randomized clinical trial. *Journal of the American Medical Association Pediatric* 171, e170698. DOI: 10.1001/jamapediatrics.2017.0698.

Martin RM, Patel R, Kramer MS, *et al.* (2013) Effects of promoting longer-term and exclusive breastfeeding on adiposity and insulin-like growth factor-I at age 11.5 years: a randomized trial. *Journal of the American Medical Association* 309, 1005–13. DOI: 10.1001/jama.2013.167. Available at: https://pubmed.ncbi.nlm.nih.gov/23483175/ (last accessed September 2022).

Martinez M (1992) Tissue levels of polyunsaturated fatty acids during early human development. *Journal of Pediatrics* 120, S129–38.

Maternal and Child Health Study Group (2013) *Maternal and Child Nutrition Series. Executive Summary of The Lancet Maternal and Child Nutrition Series.* Available at: https://www.thelancet.com/pb/assets/raw/Lancet/stories/series/nutrition-eng.pdf (last accessed August 2022).

McNeilly A (1969) Breastfeeding and the suppression of fertility. *Food and Nutrition Bulletin* 17, 163.

Modi N, Greenough A, Viner R, *et al.* for the Royal College of Paediatrics and Child Health (2017) RCPCH statement on future funding agreements with formula milk companies. *The Lancet* 389, 1693. Available at: https://www.rcpch.ac.uk/news–events/news/rcpch–statement–future–funding–agreements–formula–milk–companies/ (last accessed August 2022).

Nestlé. *Good Food, Good Life. Acting on Climate Change.* Available at: https://www.nestle.co.uk/en-gb/sustainability/climate-change (last accessed September 2022).

Neves PAR, Gatica-Domínguez G, Rollins NC, *et al.* (2020) Infant formula consumption is positively correlated with wealth, within and between countries: a multi-country study. *Journal of Nutrition* 150, 910–17.

NHS England (2017) *Managing conflicts of interest in the NHS. Guidance for staff and organizations.* Available at: https://www.england.nhs.uk/wp–content/uploads/2017/02/guidance–managing–conflicts–of–interest–nhs.pdf (last accessed August 2022).

NICE (2022) *NICE Guidance.* Available at: https://www.nice.org.uk/guidance/ (last accessed August 2022).

Odom EC, Li R, Scanlon KS, Perrine CG, Grummer-Strawn L (2013) Reasons for earlier than desired cessation of breastfeeding. *Pediatrics* 131, e726–32.

OECD (2009) *Focus on citizens: Public engagement for better policy and services.* Available at: http://www.oecd.org/governance/regulatorypolicy/focusoncitizens publicengagementforbetterpolicyandservices.htm_(last accessed August 2022).

Oken E, Patel R, Guthrie LB, *et al.* (2013) Effects of an intervention to promote breastfeeding on maternal adiposity and blood pressure at 11.5 years postpartum: results from the Promotion of Breastfeeding Intervention Trial, a cluster-randomized controlled trial. *American Journal of Clinical Nutrition* 98, 1048–56. Available at: https://pubmed.ncbi.nlm.nih.gov/23945719/ (last accessed August 2022).

PAHO (2003) *Guiding principles for complementary feeding of the breastfed child.* Available at: http://www.who.int/nutrition/publications/guiding_principles_compfeeding_breastfed.pdf (last accessed August 2022).

Panda SC (2006) Medicine: science or art? *Mens Sana Monographs* 4, 127–38.

Pinto A, Adams S, Ahring K, *et al.* (2018) Early feeding practices in infants with phenylketonuria across Europe. *Molecular Genetics and Metabolism Reports* 16, 82–89.

RCPH (2019) *RCPCH supplementary statement and FAQs on formula milk.* Available at: https://www.rcpch.ac.uk/news–events/news/rcpch–supplementary–statement–faqs–formula–milk#:~:text=On%2013%20February%202019%2C%20following,funding%20from%20formula%20milk%20companies.&text=Direct%20payments%20from%20formula%20milk,will%20no%20longer%20be%20accepted/ (last accessed August (2022).

Rosenberg BD, Siegel JT (2018) *Motivation Science* 4, 281–300.

Sankar MJ, Sinha B, Chowdhury R, *et al.* (2015) Optimal breastfeeding practices and infant and child mortality: a systematic review and meta-analysis. *Acta Paediatrica* 104S467), 3–13. DOI:10.1111/apa.13147.

Sarwar U, Nicolaou M (2012) Fraud and deceit in medical research. *Journal of Research in Medical Science* 17, 1077–81.

Save the Children (2013) *Superfood for Babies.* Available at: https://resourcecentre.savethechildren.net/document/superfood-babies-how-overcoming-barriers-breastfeeding-will-save-childrens-lives/ (last accessed July 2022).

Schroter S, Morris J, Chaudhry S, Smith, R, Barratt H (2004) Does the type of competing interest affect readers' perceptions of the credibility of research? Randomised trial. *British Medical Journal* 328, 742.

Schünemann HJ, Zhang Y, Oxman AD (2019) How to distinguish opinion from evidence in guidelines. *British Medical Journal* 366, 14606.

Schwarz EB, Brown JS, Creasman JM, *et al.* (2010) Lactation and maternal risk of type 2 diabetes: a population-based study. *American Journal of Medicine* 123, 863, e1–6. Available at: https://amjmed.org/lactation-and-maternal-risk-of-type-2-diabetes-a-population-based-study/ (last accessed August 2022).

Schwarz EB, McClure CK, Tepper PG, *et al.* (2010) Lactation and maternal measures of subclinical cardiovascular disease. *Obstetrics and Gynecology* 115(1), 41–48.

Schwarz EB, Ray RM, Stuebe AM, *et al.* (2009) Duration of lactation and risk factors for maternal cardiovascular disease. *Obstetrics and Gynecology* 113, 974–82. Available at: https://www.ncbi.nlm.nih.gov/pmc/articles/PMC2714700/ (last accessed August 2022).

Sethi BK, Chanukya GV, Nagesh VS (2016) Prolactin and cancer: has the orphan finally found a home? *Indian Journal of Endocrinology and Metabolism* 16(Suppl. S2), 195–98.

Shere H, Weijer L, Dashnow H, *et al.* (2021) Chronic lactation insufficiency is a public health issue: Commentary on 'We need patient-centered research in breastfeeding medicine' by Stuebe. *Breastfeeding Medicine* 16, 349–50. DOI: 10.1089/bfm.2021.0202.

Simmer K, Patole SK, Rao SC (2008) Long-chain polyunsaturated fatty acid supplementation in infants born at term. *Cochrane Database of Systematic Reviews* CD000376.

Singer PA, Ansett S, Sagoe-Moses I (2011) What could infant and young-child nutrition learn from sweatshops? *BMC Public Health* 11, 276.

Singh JA, Daar AS, Singer PA (2010) Shared principles of ethics for infant and young-child nutrition in the developing world. *BMC Public Health* 10, 321.

Stuebe AM, Michels KB, Willett WC, *et al.* (2009) Duration of lactation and incidence of myocardial infarction in middle to late adulthood. *American Journal of Obstetrics and Gynecology* 138, e1–e8.

UN (2018) *Levels and trends in child mortality report 2018.* Available at: https://www.un.org/en/development/desa/population/publications/mortality/child–mortality–report–2018.asp/ (last accessed August 2022).

UN (2019) *The Sustainable Development Goals Report 2019.* Available at: https://unstats.un.org/sdgs/report/2019/ (last accessed August 2022).

UNICEF (2006) *Celebrating the Innocenti Declaration on the protection, promotion and support of breastfeeding 1990–2005.* UNICEF Innocenti Research Centre.

UNICEF (2016) *From the first sign of life.* Available at: https://www.unicef.org/media/49801/file/From-the-first-hour-of-life-ENG.pdf (last accessed August 2022).

UNICEF (2021) *Infant and young-child feeding.* Available at: https://data.unicef.org/topic/nutrition/infant–and–young–child–feeding/ (last accessed August 2022).

UNICEF Baby Friendly Initiative (2020) *UNICEF UK infosheet: the provision of infant formula at food banks* (updated November 2020). Available at: https://www.unicef.org.uk/babyfriendly/wp–content/uploads/sites/2/2019/05/Provision–of–formula–milk–at–food–banks–Unicef–UK–Baby–Friendly–Initiative.pdf (last accessed August 2022).

UNICEF History. Website available at: https://www.unicef.org/history (last accessed August 2022).

United Nations Population Division (2019 Revision) *Future population growth.* Available at: https://ourworldindata.org/grapher/births–and–deaths–projected–to–2100?country=~OWID_WRL (last accessed August 2022).

van Tulleken C (2018) Overdiagnosis and industry influence: how cow's-milk protein allergy is extending the reach of infant formula manufacturers. *British Medical Journal* 363, k5056.

Velle-Forbord V, Skrastad RB, Salvesen O, *et al.* (2019) Breastfeeding and long-term maternal metabolic health in the HUNT study: a longitudinal population-based cohort study. *British Journal of Obstetrics and Gynaecology* 126, 526–34.

Victora CG, Bahl R, Barros AJD, *et al.* (2016) Breastfeeding in the 21st century: epidemiology, mechanisms, and lifelong effect. *The Lancet* 38, 475–90.

WHA (2016) *Ending inappropriate promotion of foods for infants and young children. WHA 69.9.* Available at: http://apps.who.int/gb/ebwha/pdf_files/WHA69/A69_R9–en.pdf (last accessed August 2022).

WHA (2018) *Infant and young child feeding. WHA 71.9. Agenda item 12.6 26 (May 2018).* Available at: https://apps.who.int/gb/ebwha/pdf_files/WHA71/A71_ACONF4-en.pdf (last accessed August 2022).

WHO (1981) *International Code of Marketing of Breastmilk Substitutes.* Available at: https://apps.who.int/iris/bitstream/handle/10665/40382/9241541601.pdf?sequence =1&isAllowed=y (last accessed August 2022).

WHO (1998) *Complementary feeding of young children in developing countries: a review of current scientific knowledge.* Available at: https://apps.who.int/iris/handle/10665/65932 (last accessed August 2022).

WHO (2001) Follow-up formula in the context of the International Code of Marketing of Breast-milk Substitutes. Previously available at: http://www.who.int/nutrition/follow-up_formula_eng.pdf/ (last accessed August 2022).

WHO (2001) *Report of the Expert Consultation on the optimal duration of exclusive breastfeeding.* Available at: https://apps.who.int/iris/bitstream/handle/10665/67219/WHO_NHD_01.09.pdf?ua=1 (last accessed August 2022).

WHO (2003) *Global strategy for infant and young-child feeding.* Available at: http://whqlibdoc.who.int/publications/2003/9241562218.pdf (last accessed August 2022).

WHO (2005) *Guiding principles for feeding non-breastfed children 6–24 months of age.* Available at: http://apps.who.int/iris/bitstream/handle/10665/43281/9241593431.pdf?sequence=1 (last accessed August 2022).

WHO (2006) *Constitution of the World Health Organization. Basic Documents (45th edn) Supplement.* Available at: http://www.who.int/governance/eb/who_constitution_en.pdf (last accessed August 2022).

WHO (2011) WHO Media Centre Statement, 15 January 2011. *Exclusive breastfeeding for six months best for babies everywhere.* Available at: https://www.who.int/news/item /15-01-2011-exclusive-breastfeeding-for-sixmonths-best-for-babies-everywhere(last accessed July 2022).

WHO (2012) *Supplementary foods for the management of moderate acute malnutrition in infants and children 6–59 months of age. Technical note.* Available at: https://apps. who.int/iris/handle/10665/75836 (last accessed August 2022).

WHO (2014) *Report of the Commission on Ending Childhood Obesity. Implementation plan: Executive summary.* Available at: https://apps.who.int/iris/bitstream/handle/10665/259 349/WHO–NMH–PND–ECHO–17.1–eng.pdf?sequence=1 (last accessed August 2022).

WHO (2015) *Draft clarification and guidance on inappropriate promotion of foods for infants and young children: Report of the Scientific and Technical Advisory Group (STAG) on inappropriate promotion of foods for infants and young children.* Available at: https://cdn.who.int/media/docs/default-source/nutritionlibrary/complementary -feeding/stag-report-inappropriate-promotion-infant-foods-en.pdf?sfvrsn=69120e 6a_2 (last accessed August 2022).

WHO (2015) *Sustainable Development Goals for 2030.* Available at: https://www.who. int/health-topics/sustainable-development-goals#tab=tab_1(last accessed August 2022).

WHO (2015) *WHO Secretariat response to the report of the Ebola Interim Assessment Panel.* Available at: https://www.who.int/csr/resources/publications/ebola/who-response-to-ebola-report.pdf (last accessed August 2022).

WHO (2016) *Maternal, infant, and young child nutrition. Guidance on Ending the Inappropriate Promotion of Foods for Infants and Young Children. 69th WHA Document A69/7 Add.1 2016.* Available at: http://apps.who.int/gb/ebwha/pdf_files/ WHA69/A69_7Add1-en.pdf?ua=1&ua=1/_(last accessed August 2022).

WHO (2016) *World Health Assembly resolution on the inappropriate promotion of foods for infants and young children.* Available at: https://apps.who.int/gb/ebwha/pdf_ files/WHA69/A69_R9-en.pdf?ua=1 (last accessed August 2022).

WHO (2016)*World Health Assembly resolution on the inappropriate promotion of foods for infants and young children. Policy Brief.* Available at: https://resourcecentre. savethechildren.net/pdf/WHA-Policy-brief.pdf/ (last accessed August 2022).

WHO (2017) *Approach for the prevention and management of conflicts of interest in the policy development and implementation of nutrition programmes at country level Feedback on the WHO consultation.* Available at: https://www.who.int/news-room/ events/detail/2017/09/11/default-calendar/safeguarding-against-possible-conflicts-of-interest-in-nutrition-programmes-consultation-comments (last accessed August 2022).

WHO (2017) *Guidance on Ending the Inappropriate Promotion of Foods for Infants and Young Children. Implementation manual.* Licence: CC BY-NC-SA 3.0 IGO. Available at: https://apps.who.int/iris/bitstream/handle/10665/260137/9789241513470-eng.pdf (last accessed August 2022).

WHO (2017) *Safeguarding against possible conflicts of interest in nutrition programmes.* Available at: http://apps.who.int/gb/ebwha/pdf_files/EB142/B142_23–en.pdf?ua=1 (last accessed August 2022).

WHO (2018) *Information Note. Clarification on the classification of follow-up formulas for children 6-36 months as breastmilk substitutes.* CC BY-NC-SA 3.0 IGO licence. Available at: https://apps.who.int/iris/bitstream/handle/10665/275875/WHO-NMH-NHD-18.11-eng.pdf?ua=1 (last accessed August 2022).

WHO (2019) (2016) *WHO Guideline Development Group. Meeting on complementary feeding of infants and children.* Available at: https://www.who.int/news-room/events/detail/2019/12/02/default-calendar/who-guideline-development-group-meeting-on-complementary-feeding-of-infants-and-children (last accessed August 2022).

WHO (2020) *Marketing of Breastmilk Substitutes: National Implementation of the International Code. Status Report 2020.* Available at: https://www.who.int/publications/i/item/9789240006010 (last accessed August 2022).

WHO (2021) *The optimal duration of exclusive breastfeeding. Report of an expert consultation.* Available at: https://apps.who.int/iris/bitstream/handle/10665/67219/WHO_NHD_01.09.pdf?ua=1 (last accessed August 2022).

WHO Guideline Development Group (2019) *The efficacy, safety and effectiveness of ready-to-use therapeutic foods (RUTF).* Available at: https://www.who.int/docs/default-source/blue-print/call-for-comments/2019-gdgmeeting-guideline-rutf-reduced-milkprotein-7nov-scopeandpurpose.pdf?sfvrsn=2a96a2d4_5 (last accessed August 2022).

WHO/UN Children's Fund (2017) *NetCode toolkit. Monitoring the marketing of breastmilk substitutes: protocol for ongoing monitoring systems.* Licence CC BY-NC-SA 3.0 IGO. Available at: https://apps.who.int/iris/bitstream/handle/10665/259441/9789241513180-eng.pdf (last accessed August 2022).

WHO/UNICEF (1990) *Innocenti declaration on the protection, promotion and support of breastfeeding.* Available at: https://worldbreastfeedingweek.org/2018/wp-content/uploads/2018/07/1990-Innocenti-Declaration.pdf (last accessed August 2022).

WHO/UNICEF (2003) *Global strategy for infant and young-child feeding.* Available at: http://apps.who.int/iris/bitstream/10665/42590/1/9241562218.pdf?ua=1&ua=1 (last accessed August 2022).

WHO/UNICEF (2017) *Global Breastfeeding Collective.* Available at: https://www.globalbreastfeedingcollective.org/ (last accessed August 2022).

WHO/UNICEF (2018) *Information note. Clarification on the classification of follow-up formulas for children 6–36 months as breast milk substitutes.* Available at: https://www.who.int/publications/i/item/WHO-NMH-NHD-18.11 (last accessed August 2022).

WHO/UNICEF (2021) Statement on the 40th anniversary of the *International Code of Marketing of Breastmilk Substitutes.* Available at: https://www.who.int/news/item/21-05-2021-WHO-UNICEF-statement-on-the-40th-anniversary-of-the-international-code-of-marketing-breastmilk-substitutes (last accessed August 2022).

WHO/UNICEF/IBFAN (2016) *Marketing of Breastmilk Substitutes: National Implementation of the International Code, Status Report 2016.* Available at: https://www.who.int/publications/i/item/9789241565325 (last accessed August 2022).

Willmott G, Sarbu D, Childers N, Kadenbach K (2011) Motion for a resolution pursuant to Rule 88(2) of the Rules of Procedure by Glenis Willmott, Daciana Sarbu, Nessa Childers and Karin Kadenbach on the draft commission regulation on the authorisation and refusal 000000of authorisation of certain health claims made on foods and referring to children's development and health. *European Parliament, Committee on the Environment, Public Health and Food Safety, Plenary Sitting B7 0000/2011.*

Wilson AC, Forsyth JS, Greene SA, *et al.* (1998) Relation of infant diet to childhood health: seven-year follow-up of a cohort of children in the Dundee infant feeding study. *British Medical Journal* 316, 21–25.

Wise J (2020) Food banks and infant formula: who knows best? *British Medical Journal* 371, m4449.

World Cancer Research Fund/American Institute for Cancer Research. Continuous Update Project Expert Report (2018) *Lactation and the risk of cancer.* Available at: https://www.wcrf.org/wp-content/uploads/2021/02/Lactation.pdf/ (last accessed August 2022).

Yang B, Ren XL, Fu YQ, *et al.* (2014) Ratio of *n*-3/*n*-6 PUFAs and risk of breast cancer: a meta-analysis of 274135 adult females from 11 independent prospective studies. *BMC Cancer* 14, 105.

Yang S, Martin RM, Oken E, *et al.* (2018) Breastfeeding during infancy and neurocognitive function in adolescence: 16-year follow-up of the PROBIT cluster-randomized trial. *PLoS Med* (2015), e1002554. DOI: 10.1371/journal.pmed.1002554. Available at: https://www.ncbi.nlm.nih.gov/pmc/articles/PMC5909901/ (last accessed August 2022).

Yeong JK (2014) Non-compliance with the *International Code of Marketing of Breastmilk Substitutes* is not confined to the infant-formula industry. *Public Health (Oxf)* 2014, 352, 193–94. DOI: 10.1093/pubmed/fdt026/). Available at: https://pubmed.ncbi.nlm.nih.gov/23564839/ (last accessed August 2022).

Useful links

Access to Nutrition Index (ANI)
www.accesstonutrition.org

Agency for Healthcare Research and Quality (US) (AHRQ)
www.ahrq.gov

Baby Friendly Initiative (BFI)
www.unicef.org.uk/babyfriendly

Baby Milk Action
www.babymilkaction.org

Baby-Friendly Hospital Initiative (BFHI)
www.unicef.org/documents/baby-friendly-hospital-initiative

Codex Alimentarius International Food Standards
www.fao.org

UN Economic and Social Council (ECOSOC)
www.un.org/ecosoc

Effective Health Care (EHC)
www.effectivehealthcare.ahrq.gov

European Academy of Paediatrics (EAP)
www.eapaediatrics.eu

European Food Safety Authority (EFSA)
www.efsa.europa.eu

European Society for Paediatric Gastroenterology, Hepatology and Nutrition
(ESPGHAN)
www.espghan.org

European Society for Paediatric Infectious Diseases (ESPID)
www.espid.org

European Society for Paediatric Nephrology (ESPN)
www.espn-online.org

European Society for Paediatric Research (ESPR)
www.espr.eu

European Society of Emergency Medicine (EUSEM)
www.eusem.org

European Society of Paediatric and Neonatal Intensive Care (ESPNIC)
www.espnic.eu

Food Administration Organization (FAO)
www.fao.org

Global Alliance for Improved Nutrition (GAIN)
www.gainhealth.org

Global Breastfeeding Collective
www.globalbreastfeedingcollective.org

Infant Feeding Action Coalition (INFACT)
www.infactcanada.ca

Interagency Group on Breastfeeding Monitoring (IGBM)
https://uia.org/s/or/en/1100050028

International Baby Food Action Network (IBFAN)
www.ibfan.org

International Labour Organization (ILO)
www.ilo.org/global

International Life Sciences Institute (ILSI)
www.ilsi.org

The Lives Saved Tool
www.livessavedtool.org

Nestlé UK
www.nestle.co.uk

Organization for Economic Cooperation and Development (OECD)
www.oecd.org

Index